Lil' Lymie Fly Away Home

By Nicolenya Caltman

Table of Contents

Dedication

For my adorable, beautiful, man…my dearest darling. I could not have voyaged the green sea without you, and "M" who held me up and kept me from falling. My daughters Julie and Jackie, grandchildren Lilly, Elsie, NayNay, Tobyas, Leila, My sons Micaiah and Ivan, and Mason even though he can't deal with me with this disease right now, my mom, and Rosie…and Merriam-Webster, who always seems to have just the right definitions for me! (All definitions are property of Merriam-Webster.com and Verses from KJV.)

Introduction

Welcome to my suffering. I am Nicolenya. I have Lyme. Sounds like an opening for a support group…but there it is. I am beginning to think that much like the saying "Once an alcoholic, always an alcoholic" is true in this case, and that in my case "Once a "Lymie", always a "Lymie" will be my lot. I don't want to believe it but I fear this is the path I am going down. There really should be support groups all over the world for us and beautiful retreats to run away to, where we can receive love and encouragement…but there isn't…perhaps someday. A beautiful, novel, idea.

I decided to try to write this book with the hope that in reading about my suffering, it will alleviate yours some…that you won't feel so alone in the "Green Sea"…that someone is suffering in spirit with you and holding your hand in bed…and that a most delicate, intimacy will be shared…and through our "communion of souls" we can make it through this together. I should forewarn you, there is a lot of cussing in here…it is not meant to offend…and I have a feeling anyone with this disease has at least thought the words in their head. LOL

I hope that somehow this book will also help to shift the beliefs of the "standard medical community and insurances". That they will all start to look better at this little-known disease (even though it has been around for eons), and realize it is quickly turning into a pandemic issue capable of epic proportions…and start taking it seriously.

I am writing this in the middle of yet another relapse to keep myself from wanting to jump off a cliff into a beautiful, deep, canyon of rocks and hoping that all my suffering will have not been all for naught…and that somehow it will turn into a miracle that saves someone else from suffering the devastating effects of Lyme. Even if the miracle oil comes from sarcastic laughter at my "groanings" in our shared experience.

The exercises I have included in this book are strategically placed through out to give us time to really take time on our healing and coming home to ourselves. Take note that these exercises are geared at "spirituality" and not religion. I however have made references from the Bible in there in case there are those out there who question because they might be Christian they shouldn't do them. I myself am a "Christian". I believe in love. I believe God would want us to be perfect and whole.

There will be a lot of back and forth as I go through this healing with you. I am 47 years old and have taught classes on spirituality for over 20 years. The methods in this book are created by me at the request of clients both privately and in classes I have taught; "Isn't there an easier way?". I personally have seen quick changes for people in doing them. It is my hope that somehow, they will help us find peace in the middle of the "green sea".

My best advice for other "Lymies" out there…do not wait for someone else to be your advocate. Be your own, and research like a mad man…and above all, don't give up…"Nik"

Chapter 1

The Worst Death of All~The Death of The Self

I want to die. I do. I am done. I am done with this mother fucking disease. I am angry, and barely holding on to my sanity. I have lost almost everything to this disease. My new small, but useful career as a personal trainer and belly dance-fitness instructor after working diligently losing 248 pounds…my body, gaining back about 60 of it from damage done to my thyroid and my poor body and not being to exercise…members of my family…almost lost my boyfriend several times I think he's still here…and the worst death of all…the death of myself. The beautiful self I found after my beautiful divorce, after losing myself temporarily to that "ass hat"…I am still trying to forgive.

There has been such a waste of time with my health, between not having the right family support, the right doctors, doctors not listening to me and just thinking I am crazy. When the reality of it I am probably saner than them. I am more aware than them…shame on them. Shame on them for making me think I was crazy! My life, your life is worth something…and we deserve to be helped.

I am tired of these sleepless nights. I take enough Melatonin to knock down a rhino (about 20 tonight) and here I am up. I am tired of the crying, of the hurting, and feeling like an "untouchable" in India. I hate looking at myself in the mirror after working so hard to love my body, elephant skin and all. To go from a woman unashamed to show her belly while dancing to a woman who just wants to crawl in a hole…disgusts me. I hate myself. Which is a problem, because I look for acceptance from my boyfriend. I am aware of my shortcomings since Lyme and it makes me hate myself even more. I don't feel like a woman. I feel more like a frumpy, dumpy, curmudgeon, ogre type thingy hiding in a hole. I have become a recluse.

Is it so bad to need him to just grab me, throw me on the bed, and ravage me like a burly pirate, pillage and plunder the gems of the ruby fruits…and make me feel like a woman again? His very own private little tart? Hot pocket? One doesn't feel sexy in the act of glorious self-love…Oh yes, by the way...I have been failing to orgasm. Lyme has apparently taken that from me too. Did you know that can happen? I'd like to believe it is just because it has been WAY TOO LONG!!! However, I don't think that is so. Others out there have spoken of the same experience.

I feel so out of sync with myself and the world around me. I miss dancing, teaching, supporting, sex with my boyfriend, sex with my boyfriend. Yes, I said it twice. I miss feeling sexy, I miss feeling and being strong. I miss kettlebells. Where did I go? How do I find myself again? Sex with my BOYFRIEND would be an awesome place to start. It however is just a guilty pleasure and doesn't fix what's wrong inside of me. The truth is I don't know I could get naked in front of him right now even if he were here. I feel so gross and unappealing. My beautiful self is hidden somewhere deep inside of me and I am scared I'll never find her again from the filthy little buggers using my brain like a cafeteria.

I know I should be meditating. I was a spiritual teacher as well. It isn't that easy to get quiet and meditate when you have millions of minions milling around in your brain digging for gold…your gold…your gems. Your intelligence, your creativity, your voice, your truth. I had a high IQ before, it is mediocre at best now. I have shitty short-term memory, my impulse control sucks ask my boyfriend, and now it has begun to affect my long-term memory. I can't do math past fractions now, misspelling words, forget what I am doing, what I am saying, it has affected my speech at times so bad no one can understand me, I still stutter at times so FUCKING EMBARASSING and at random times…never knowing when it is going to come out.

I am scared to death to even have sex with my boyfriend at this point. I am very verbal with him and it makes me cry even now as I write this. Can you imagine? "OOOH YYYES BBBBABY PPPPOKE IIIIT RRRIGHT TTTTHERE" Oh hell no! I'd rather be gagged. While I am sure my boyfriend would be very gracious, understanding, and beautiful because that's who he is, I just can't even fathom the thought.

It has affected my already suffering penmanship and overnight. My one pleasure right now in the midst of all this is all the art painting and clay I do for my darling. Poor dear. He humors me with it. It is starting to look like the "Wall of Gaylord" at my house…At one point I could barely do anything for him and I thought I would just die.

I fell five maybe six times last year. Was walking so bad at one point the hospital staff kept trying to shove a walker down my throat. I'd rather die. I refused. I am a very difficult patient. Can't keep me down. I am very rough on my body. I am so used to having been independent my whole life and was such a beast exercising before this has been a very huge pill to swallow. The woman who needed no epidural during birth, up and walking right after C-sections, gallbladder surgery, and walked a mile in the hospital after a hysterectomy (also Lyme related)…now pretty much glued to the couch or my bed.

I try to push myself but walking is very hard for me now. I have tried dancing before months earlier but had issues after and well, quite honestly…I am afraid of failing again and haven't tried.

My body is so depleted of vital nutrients from the minions who knows whether how I feel is related to lack of nutrients and actually in remission or if I am still infected. No one will test me or help me. I did finally get help from one doctor who could sympathize with me and tried but she was a traveling doctor and left. There has been nobody since.

Constant denial, and why? I have late stage chronic Lyme. Yes, that's right…Even

infectious disease doctors denying me for the same reason. Handfuls of them. Like they

are just washing their hands of me. I do have an appointment finally not for six weeks

and because a referral wasn't filled out right.

Then there are the "LLMDs" Lyme literate medical doctors; who charge an

astronomical fee that people must go in debt for emptying their savings, using charge

cards to pay because insurance companies won't cover Lyme visits, or tests. People like

me can't afford the illustrious chosen ones because they charge about $1,000 for the first

visit. Who knows how much for the rest.

I want to give up…but I promised my boyfriend I would keep fighting.

It has been about three weeks since I have been off the antibiotics. I went off at two

and a half months after round four because of what they were doing to my brain. Scary

things…bump in the night things. Things I haven't spoken of to anyone except the insurance company out of necessity…not even my boyfriend. I started going through "episodes" of violent rocking, hitting my head, feeling like bugs were crawling on me, up down, up down I went on the bed, restless legs…just to name a few. It went on for several hours the first time. All night. The other two were slightly less time but the same effect. Very exorcist like.

Each time losing another ability and piece to myself. However, there was a welcomed change after the first episode. I had been in horrific pain I can't even describe. Think elephant sitting on your lower extremities and playing Twister. The night before the episode I had horrific pain and after no pain. None. Not normal. Probably from brain damage. Little by little I do seem to have more pain sensation creeping back but not like before. Very minimal.

I have tried everything. So many antibiotics, supplements and natural remedies. They would work in the start of them only to go back to the same vicious circle. This is because as I found out later, the Lyme bacteria can morph into cysts and in and out when they feel threatened and then one feels better seemingly. Then suddenly, its sudden death match…and they multiply. They are angry and you get sicker it seems each time. The bacteria essentially fart as they are dying creating a noxious gas you can't get rid of…neurotoxins. Just as difficult to chase. If you try to detox through sweating which is supposed to be the best, you must take a long hot shower right away or it gets soaked right back into your body and can create rashes and sores on your skin. This has been my problem. I live in a house with almost my whole family.   There are seven people all living in my mother's house. So, she understandably so watches the bills. We all pay a section but still showers are a problem. As it is I take a shower about every three days at about 5 minutes is the allowance. If I exercised etc. It would be a huge problem because I couldn't get the toxins off me. Who knows if I could even dance etc. again anyway.

I have so much belly dance gear it looks like I pooped coins and glitter everywhere. I yearn to get into my garb again. I feel its calling to wear the baubles and bangles deep within my soul. The sadness growing within me is epic, missing my dance. Am I the greatest dancer? Laughing, no! It feeds me though and I have seen worse.

It's like my inspiration is gone. The only inspiration I seem to have is the deep love I have for my darling, that forces out a cacophony of chaos and color likened to a pooping pegacorn. In all my arting, farting for him I have found a part of myself I lost long ago...a feeling of joyful, childlike, innocence and mysticism that is as overwhelming for me as I am sure it is to him. If I lost my ability to art and fart around for him…I think I would die inside. What then would I have to give him but just a jumbled mass of blek?

This is very hard to share all of this of myself. I hope it helps you somehow feel a little less alone in reading.

I am hanging on by a thread and about to have a break down. It would not take much more to push me over the edge. I wish there were some sort of Lyme support group out there or even online. There are some out there but minimal and I have never gotten answers. They all seem to be old bulletin boards where there is no life. Probably because everyone there is suffering too. I have thought of starting one myself but again I am like you…tired and run down. Sometimes though the greatest supporters are the ones who need supporting. So, we will see what I do with this thought.

I am tired of feeling this neurotic mess inside my head and so worried I'll lose my boyfriend to this because it is hard to handle. I can't see one reason why he is even still with me at the moment; and consider myself a very lucky woman. Without him, my inspiration to any goodness within myself…I have lost so much of myself through this disease, I would wither and die. Herein lies my problem. Because of this disease in my brain now I think obsessively so about losing him because of my mess with this disease. If I lost my ability to art for him, and write poetry for him; it is how I express love for him…I would have nothing to offer him anymore and all he would be left with is this shell of a person. So, I spew out from my soul as much love as I can possibly art so he has a record of sorts of how important and precious he is to me in case I run out of time and words to love him. I am not good at expressing in person the love I have inside me for people because I have not had a lot of it myself in life. Just since him.

The last few episodes were really, hard on me. I am afraid to go to sleep because I might not wake up and be able to love my son or my darling anymore or my kids who still love me regardless of what I can do for them from this disease…or my grandkids. I am so tired I can barely see straight at this point. This book is my last effort to re-channel my energy somehow and try to make this fucking disease count for something…that the knowledge that others are not alone in their struggle will somehow comfort them and perhaps this doctor will be able to cure me and then I can share the wealth of info with others and in the process of this won't drive my boyfriend crazy.

Perhaps my amazing will be shown…so that I can find myself again and then become a compliment to him and my family so that I don't feel like an albatross around their necks…a burden. Members of my family have called me a burden since this disease…but My Darling never has. Even though I have been a huge pain in his ass whether I could help it or not…he's been there and never not even once called me a burden; and when I am not in the midst of minions eating my brain he helps me to see I have something to offer the world. I have gotten sidetracked though at times because of the debilitating pain, the "misfiring" in my brain that is always unexpected, and then just the unwieldy weight that having this disease carries.

I wonder if I will ever be able to rise above this. Sometimes it is just too much. According to the statistics the death rate is not high for Lyme for health reasons though can happen; the death rate is very high among our fellow "Lymie's" due to suicide. My heart goes out to all of you who are thinking about this. I can understand. I hate being in this body and I have at times wished I would just die and not wake up; because so much

of myself was lost, coupled with the lack of support, then the pain was just too much to

bare. I was very afraid this was going to make me insane.

If you were drawn to this book there is a reason. There is help out there for you and

me. We just have to continue to forge forward and refuse to let Lyme define us or defeat

us. We all need to ban together, and help each other find our balance again.

Throughout the course of this book you will notice I have many bad days as I go

through the healing process. I am daring to bear all for you so that you do not feel alone

in this, feel ostracized, untouchable; abnormal. Will I come out of this okay? It is a

mystery. However, whether I come out of this or not…doesn't mean you couldn't. Each

body is different, you just have to keep trying. What worked for some won't work for

others and yet there will be something that might work. Through the "Lymie" grapevine a

solution could be there for you and it is worth everything to try one day at a time to find

out. You owe that to yourself for weathering the "Green Sea" like you have.

It is important for all of us to find an outlet both creative and societal in nature, even if that society is online temporarily and encourage each other so we don't feel so alone in this. I know firsthand what it's like to feel like hiding in a cave and just cutting yourself off. I have gained a lot of weight, lost a lot of hair, not had a lot of support and I am tired and spent. As I sit here writing this I am just disgusted with the degenerating mess that appears before me. I know many of you feel the same, and perhaps we can help each other find that inner light that I know is there somewhere and exemplify each other's beauty. You are beautiful and worthy of receiving healing, love, and support.

Who knows what I will be like later today. I go through many spurts of changes during the day. It changes day to day. I hope to be able to remain committed to our cause so that somehow, in some way together we can make Lyme Disease a thing of the past.

Chapter 2

The Art of Letting Go~Clearing the Thicket and Our Path To Our Healing

Well today not doing so good with this subject. I can't seem to get past all my anger around this and how much I have lost. I have ostracized myself to my room because I just can't handle my family right now. The loud noises and lack of disrespect is making my head spin, and I just want to cry in my room to try to get it out as I attempt to continue to write this book. At least regardless of my upset I have been able to give my boyfriend some space and not hold on too tight for the moment.

My darling, is just so lovely to love. I love big though. To someone who hasn't had much of it, it can be overwhelming. Like it was to me at first when we met. I had a very hard time letting him in…letting go of the past enough to fall in love with him…but that man did it. Not only did he get some of my love…he got the whole stinkin' lot of it. Now the roles are reversed I guess. HaHa. All I want to do is fucking shower him with glitter bombs of love, and not let him come up for air from making love to him…I want to freaking "Fockerize" him like he did me…climb up and down his walls…what's fair is fair.

However, I think I need to cool it a bit on the fire I have for him and the towering "Wall Of Gaylord" building up and let go just a little. It's hard because never in my life have a met a man with so much charisma, and saucy sexiness, then he is just so sweet besides.

I am referring to him a lot in this book because this has been such a challenge for me since the Lyme and losing a lot of my brain that has that impulse control. For others, you might have other challenges. For me this is the "big un", I have so much love for him, so much oh my gawd…want, desire, and attraction for him and with not a lot of impulse control I could give the poor man a coronary. In one of our saucy sessions, he actually had to tell me to slow down because I was breathing too hard (I could have burned his clothes right off his body as hot as I was). I just wanted grab him and UHHH! LOL Damned man anyway. LOL.

For you, perhaps you are holding on to your family too tight or people, places, things, and our disease. What a word "eh"? Just for my Canadian friend. DISEASE…sounds delicious I know. Let's break it down though:

Compliments of Google Search:

Their definition is perfect for this.

"a disorder of structure or function in a human, animal, or plant, especially one that produces specific signs or symptoms or that affects a specific location and is not simply a direct result of physical injury."

"A disorder of structure that is not a direct result of physical injury". If there is no direct result, that means it just "appeared" out of nowhere. Perhaps, and I know with my spiritual training…I manifested this. Any disease within the body has a lot to do with a deep-rooted regret and anger…whether at someone else or ourselves.

I have had a lot of different and strange ailments I have healed myself from just from dealing with certain emotions or paying attention to what I am not doing for myself. I healed from a heart condition I was told I would always take medicine for, a rare brain issue that went into "remission" for twenty years in which I almost lost my eye site, among other smaller nuisances.

I am very rough on my body as I said before and myself. As a teenager and for good reason I had a lot of anger inside of me from being raped when I was ten and not receiving any support for it and many other things that just seemed to pile on. I saw crying as a sign of weakness and stuffed things down. It took a long time for me to figure out how to at least manage the anger. It was still there though. I still never cried. There was still a lot there; to cry about.

Later, I was fortunate to find these beautiful people who helped me begin the healing process inside of me. This is when these other ailments left. Then I get myself in this piss poor marriage. I started getting very angry at him, at myself because I was afraid to leave and that I had allowed his abuse to go on and was stupid enough to marry him.

The one thing that started to become clear during this stupid disease, is that once it got

into my brain and did something to my impulse control, I couldn't hang on to stuff

anymore without also releasing in tears. Forgiveness, actually became easier than it ever

was…and it became even easier for me to love. I always loved people…especially when I

was a little girl. I however don't ever remember loving myself. I remember as a child

watching paper and trash fly around on the ground and thinking to myself I am no better

than that trash. Even at about three years old. I thought I was nothing but waste.

I know all these principles, yet I am still angry at this situation and what I have lost. I

am really struggling with it and know I must let it go so I can really enjoy my life and

really enjoy loving my boyfriend. Gawd help the man when I fall in love with myself.

LOL This is my new goal and my goal for you.

You might be saying, "So, you are telling us that all we have to do is the bullshit;

think and it is?" No. I am only saying it is an aspect of it and should be utilized in our

path of healing from these stupid medications we must take, because the medicines can

cause other issues and we need the inner strength to fight this. They have done studies on

this type of thing and even Cancer Treatment Centers of America, focus also on meditation and the self. So, I have chosen to get back to my roots, and I encourage you to join me.

As I stated before I was a spiritual teacher and taught meditation to numerous clients privately and in classes, including children. I will be including exercises throughout this book for you to begin on this journey of healing with me, and encourage you to not just stay within these exercises just using them as a beginning foundation to the new you. Starting the first exercise on a new page. Just a thing I have. LOL.

KEY: 1 READINESS-

Step1. Clearing the Thicket:

Thicket-2: something resembling a thicket in density or impenetrability.

When we have experienced what is to some a lot of drama in our lives, and we haven't been able to work on it for whatever reason, it makes the area around our person very dense and impenetrable. Many don't even know where to begin in this process and it is why I chose to share this with you. There is both good and what I will call alternative news.

The good news: By the end of this step if you follow precisely in my direction, you will begin to feel liberated and things will be transforming all around you I promise.

The alternative: It is also the most difficult for people to overcome and move forward to their new life and way of living.

However, I know you can do it. I have faith in you.

Step1. Acknowledgment

The first step in clearing the thicket is acknowledgment. Acknowledgment at whatever you might not be at peace with, i.e. your love life, body, job...what vexes you the most? People don't like to pay attention to what is not working for them. It is perhaps the most crucial step, and is usually the easiest.

You might say, "Nothing is vexing me. I love my job, my boss, have a wonderful, mate...somehow I still am not peaceful." Well, I say to you then there is something vexing you. Perhaps that vexes you, that you aren't peaceful, that you aren't satisfied with your life.

Get out your notebook and write down in list form:

I am vexed by:

1. No boy friend

2. Love job, hate boss

These are just examples. The point is you need to be very specific. Like number two for instance...you may love your job, but hate your boss. So don't just put hate job. Take your time on this about a week.

Step2. Forgiveness:

Now, here is where a lot of people get frustrated and lost. There however, is more good news you only must forgive one person. I am sure I really have you going now. You are probably wondering but, So and So did this and that to me. You need to understand that one person the only one you need to forgive is yourself. Let me explain:

Before we come into this world we are given a few, even several choices at what type of life we desire to live. Even the Bible speaks of predestination. We are given the opportunity to design our lives. We choose people to be our parents, friends, etc. to help us learn lessons for further evolvement. Nothing is by chance. I was once where you were at. In fact, I may have even been in a worse place. I used to make more excuses why I couldn't do this and that. This person and that person did that and this to me. Though it is true I have experienced things in my life most would consider traumatic, I now understand I chose to experience those things and I now give thanks for the lessons I have learned.

I will never forget the day I was meditating…my effort to "escape" when I started crying uncontrollably. I was raising my fists toward the sky, toward God…WHY? WHY?…You know, the poor me deal. I was crying, sobbing, "I can't take this anymore. Give me a way out." Then I sort of heard this whisper from within myself, "Forgiveness is the only way, not forgiveness of others, forgiveness of yourself." Was my answer. Oh my, this response did not go over well with me.

Then instead of cursing God I was cursing myself. You know…the whole "What is wrong with you deal. Can't you do anything right"? I spoke words against myself with such fervor…and of course I did it in front of the mirror even better, all of it reflecting; back to me. I doubled over with writhing pain in my abdomen.

Then it happened. I wept and wept and wept. Suddenly I got it…it all made sense. I shrugged my shoulders, figured what do I have to lose? I decided I was ready to try to allow God to really start working with me and that I was no longer going to fight it.

Now, before you start thinking…here we go another "hippie dippie" another "bible thumper"…I have boxing rounds with God. I get pissed and have even flipped God off.

Not my finest moments. What I know about God just from my own life is that this loving presence meets you where you are at. Currently I am pretty; pissed. I feel abandoned by God…this presence that is supposed to love me and protect me. This God; however, has a sense of humor and I suppose this book is his/her/its way of saying I haven't left.

So, when I wrote this exercise I was recollecting one very pivotal and unmistakable moment in my life. I began to speak to "GOD".

"God, if you are there…(notice my choice of words) please love me show me your love because I don't know how to love myself."

In a nano second, I felt so much almost overwhelming unconditional love. It was then that I realized that if God has so much love for me surely, I can love myself. I began to forgive myself, forgiving myself for relinquishing my power and creating all the mess.

Almost immediately things started changing. More money was coming in, even money from unexpected resources. My relationships improved, even relationships thought to be over.

Most importantly, I started to love myself. Each day, I looked at myself in the mirror and told myself how much I love you, (me). I focused on the gifts and talents I have. I began to lose weight without even trying or dieting. I began to be grateful for everything I had in my life even the difficult lessons I created for myself. I however never fell in love with myself. This is now my journey. Please join me.

It is time for you to work on forgiving yourself as well.

Get out your notebook:

Write.

Ex. I forgive myself for giving up my power to others…

I forgive myself for…Be careful not to place blame on others.

Really try to pay attention to what starts happening in your body. Allow emotion to come. No stuffing. We aren't turkeys. You may find that going to a healer or minister might be beneficial or even confession but is not necessary. Be mindful if you do go to a healer choose them carefully, and do not become dependent. I have gone to healers myself multiple times. It can be a very beneficial and beautiful experience. I had to learn though how to maintain this myself. Something always seemed to be missing. It was then that I asked God to work with me. You can do the same thing…ask God, Spirit, the Holy Father, Jesus, whoever it is to you, to pour down through you the light, to pour through you, that unconditional love. You'll feel it. UNDOUBTEDLY…Just be open.

Step3. Loving of The Self

It is best to work on this receiving love from God for at least a week. At that point I would like you to get out your notebook and begin to write:

"I love myself because"…

Come up with at least a page. I think it will be easier at this stage than you may think. Once you have your page done (more is fine), it is time to move to step 4.

Step4. I Am Affirmations

Your "I am's" are very important because you are affirming your love for yourself and how great you are. This is a very powerful process. Make this sacred Perhaps you would like to set up some candles and incense, or do your "I am's" in the park with nature.

Point being…make a sacred space.

1. Breathe in your nose and out your mouth, (breathing through your diaphragm) slowly and deliberately releasing any negativity you may have from your day.

Repeat 5x.

2. Breathe in your nose and out your nose again breathing from your diaphragm. Breathe as slow as is comfortable.

Repeat 5x.

Now it is time to start in with your affirmations. Keeping your eyes closed begin. Do not look at your list. Do the ones that simply come to mind first.

Say like this: I am beautiful. (ex.) I am beautiful.

You can say them out loud or to yourself. What counts is that you state them with conviction. When you state your affirmations really get into the feeling of it all. Repeat them as many times as you feel the need.

Step 5. Gratitude's

Gratitude's are probably one of the most interesting phenomenon's in my book. You would be surprised at the swiftness of things turning around just by stating how grateful you are for the things around you. This isn't because God wishes to hear gratitude. God has no needs because God is perfect balance. It was a blessed gift God gave us to help us acknowledge the beauty in our lives. When we are in a state of gratitude we are in total splendor of the beauty around us. To be in this state is likened to being in love. Love transforms, and transcends all.

What are you grateful for? Perhaps it is your child, or a child…or a pet? Perhaps it is the green grass or that you are able to see the green grass.

1. Become aware of what you are grateful are. Make a list.

2. Get involved with your list. Really feel the gratitude for your child, your pet, or

the grass. Get wrapped up in the beauty, feel it from your heart center. Most of us have been in love before it is the same thing. Fall in love with the beauty around you. Fall in love with every intricate quality of the grass, of your pet, of your child. Think of how miraculous that all this was created from something of such a microscopic size…Or if you can wrap your mind around that it was all created with a thought of beauty from God. That God created the cells that make us. Our DNA…Careful, deliberate, thought went into creating us and the grass, seeds, animals, the sky. Everything serves a purpose. Everything has a place…Everything is important. Everything matters…Including you.

Be grateful for you. God is.

Step 6. Discernment and Speaking with God.

God speaks to everyone. We; as a society, are usually too busy to take the time out to listen. It is easier than you may think. All it takes is the willingness to slow down, to breathe and then just simply God will speak to you. Divine (information you can trust) knowledge comes from the right-hand side. Our ego and where alternative energies try to get to us at times come from the left. Divine knowledge always has a loving edge, always no exception. Do not confuse this with loving…being what we want to do. Say you want to do something, or go somewhere but you are hesitating. It may not be safe for you to go…pay close attention. Sometimes it will be loud, sometimes a whisper or even a thought. Just because you "get" you shouldn't go…   from the right doesn't mean it's not loving. You will get a message something like it is not in your best interest to go at this time.

Something from the left hand side would sound like this…"You don't deserve to go". If you are hearing negativity or negative thoughts it is the left no question. It may be coming close, very close to the right and this is where you really have to quiet the mind to pay attention where it is really coming from. To be aware of this difference do the following.

Begin by again breathing as mentioned previously.

1. Breathe in your nose and out your mouth, (breathing through your diaphragm) slowly and deliberately releasing any negativity you may have from your day.

Repeat 5x.

2. Breathe in your nose and out your nose again breathing from your diaphragm. Breathe as slow as is comfortable.

Repeat 5x.

Place your index and middle finger together in the middle of your forehead. After a couple of minutes, you will start to feel a shift and be aware of the difference. Once you feel this, remove your fingers and begin to shift attention to right, then left, right, left…getting quicker and quicker until the awareness is there of the split, but you don't need to go back and forth…where it "just is". If your info is from the right it is "Divine" info you can trust…if the left, ego and conditioning.

Practice this about a week or so and really spend some time getting acquainted with God, maybe even your higher self, and your angels. When you feel like you have this concept down move forward to Step 7.

Step 7. FUN

I figured that would get your attention. If you have gotten this far you should be proud of yourself. You deserve a little fun.

It is time to start acknowledging your needs. What is it you wish for? Love? Money? Health? We aren't getting into specifics here. That will come later.

Make your list. Take your time on this. Spend about a week on it.

1. I wish for love in my life. (for example)

2. I wish for a new car (we aren't getting into the make or model here. Just the wishing for now. This is just simply acknowledging.)

Do not limit your thinking on this. The sky is the limit. Write down everything, and again take your time. When you feel you have completed this and you no longer wish for anything move on to the next KEY.

I am awake again. So, I go back to read what I have written and get to the part where it mentions FUN. I am doing these exercises along with you…and I just have to say this disease is not fucking fun! I am so sick of waking up at odd hours, not getting sleep, sores in my nose, shaking, tremors, dry eyes, stiffness, thick mucus in my throat that makes me gag (how freakin' sexy is that?), the feeling of BLAH, the feeling of dread, constant body temp changes, blood sugar drops, feeling like somethings eating my brain, heart racing, bla, bla, bla,. Stupid MOFO disease! I am so fucking sick of it.

I feel like just smoking a huge bag of that sweet Mary Jane and going WWII on the filthy buggers, even though it would tear up my lungs. Smoke the fuckers out. FUCK ME! Will I ever be normal again!!!??? Ok, ok, I have never really been normal…LOL but the normal me…Ya' know? I feel like sucking down a grenade and BOOM! BOOM! No more Lyme! VOILA!…Fuckers…blimey, mother fucking, fuckers.

Sighing…

See? I am human. I am spiritual, but I am also human…and I am tired. I don't know what I am going to do if this nonsense doesn't stop. Not doing a very good job letting go right now, am I? This is why, I am writing this book though. Perhaps you are up right now too reading this and at your end, and now we are up together…and you are not alone.

Something, I have seen a lot are people getting stuck in the how's of it all. How in the hell did I even get this? I know I have. Was it the fawn, horse, or pea chick I rescued? Was it the man who raped me when I was 10…How long have I even had this? How long has my body been sick? How am I going to get this to stop and out of my body? One can how them self to death…and it ultimately doesn't matter does it? We just have to figure out a way to stop going around in circles so we can fight this…and this is why I am including the exercises. I am unsure if it will even help me at this stage because I have a lot of brain damage. I have to try something though. Even if it didn't, and it helped you…then my darling…this journey was all worth it.

;-)

Chapter 3

Falling in Love with Yourself~Realizing You Are Deserving of Great Good

Since the Lyme hit, I have been so hateful towards myself and constant with it. Lyme has turned me into someone I do not like at all; so much so I have abandoned myself. I woke up at 3 AM today and immediately started crying. Instead of being kind to myself, I immediately say "What the fucking fuck; is wrong with you?!". I go to the bathroom, sit on the toilet…I notice I am rocking. Now I am bawling. "NO! NO! NO! I can't go through another one of these episodes! NO! I am not doing this! Not today. You cannot have my body anymore as a fucking waste hole for you to crap in!"

I fix myself a nice hot cup of coffee (which can tend to make matters worse FYI) go back to my room, get out my computer, put on Myrica Faya (a beautiful Portuguese band, no I don't understand them…), and light some incense (Nag Champa. You should try it its nice and mellow)…and start writing to you. I have decided to consider this book love letters to you. I have felt such a lack of love since this disease. I really have not had great support from my family. My mom has done better lately. My older adult children still haven't respected my need for rest, or how sick I really am.

My 16-year-old son Ivan has been really great. The dear boy has massaged me repeatedly to ease my pain and relax me. He is 16 though and shouldn't have this responsibility on him, which makes me feel like shit. I really don't know what I would have done without him and my boyfriend who even when it hasn't been convenient, even when I was acting like a mad woman, has chosen to support me, and show love for me anyway. That I was still; worthy of love, still sexy…even though I was breaking down. I know though, all the love can't come from him. I know this. My soul just can't seem to connect very well to my brain anymore. There is a direct correlation between the brain and the soul. Somehow, I have to find that connection again.

I am great at showing love to others but not to myself. Myself has always been a problem…but I did find it for a time. I feel sometimes, almost like my soul has disconnected from my body in a very similar way to those who are unconscious; because my soul which is strong and loving can't relate to this decaying body…and I somehow have to connect back to my soul and get it flowing back through me again because it is the only thing that might save me with this. It is why I have made exercises a part of this book. To keep us connected to our soul which is beautifully strong and loving so we can somehow beat this. I know others with this disease have gone through the same thing in respect to feeling separate from others and themselves and haven't felt love and support in dealing with this disease and is what has driven them to suicide. I want to change this somehow for all of us…so that when we all feel like giving up…in the times we can't get help from doctors, family, or ourselves…remember in that very minute…when you feel your most defeated…and even though we don't know each other…that I love you.

I don't know if all these things I am having issues with right now is just damage done to my brain now or if I am still infected. How am I supposed to find out when I can't get help? My brain is off today; really bad. I am having issues writing and typing even as I write to this now to you.

Right when I was taking a break from writing for today, I had a major epiphany that went with this chapter. I realized I don't feel worthy and deserving of my boyfriend because I am so fucked up right now. That in my head, I feel he is so much more deserving than the broken-down woman I am right now. I am trying to put myself back together while I am waiting for the doctor appointment, but I am really

going through another bad phase right now and I am not perfect. That is going to have to be okay with me. I have had a huge fight treading a terrible "green sea"…I have had a lot of smelly, sour, lemons in my life and I deserve good…good like him good. He smells so sweet, deliciously musky, his kisses are divine, and he is most definitely not sour and is the sweetest most adorable man I have ever known. I do deserve an amazing man like him because I am a good woman. I am not going to be perfect no one is and I just need to find a way to deal with the lack I am feeling within myself.

I am sure I am going to have lots of off days as I continue writing this book as you will see. This was huge though. I know there are others out there in the same situation…feeling just like jumping ship. This is a debilitating, terrible, mother fucking, asshole of a disease. We can do this though.

Before we fall in love with ourselves, we first have to learn to accept ourselves…and this is the next KEY.

KEY: 2 ACCEPTANCE-

Acceptance 2: the quality or state of being accepted or acceptable 3: the act of accepting; the fact of being accepted: approval

Being-1 a: the quality or state of having existence b (1): something conceivable as existing (2): something that actually exists 3: a living thing;

(Merriam-Webster)

Here you'll notice two definitions. I did this because acceptance had a very important word in it…BEING. The two words go together and have everything to do with love…which is a living thing.

Step1. Feeding the Self

Feeding of the self is essential if you are to receive great good. What is it you are not doing for yourself? It may be something you used to do and stopped doing, or perhaps something new you would like to do but are ignoring your desire. If you are giving yourself lack, if you are not honoring your needs and deepest desires, how can you expect to receive blessings or healing you if you are in a constant state of self-punishment and self-loathing? If you know of certain things to help keep you balanced and you aren't doing them, or if you are ignoring things you know you should be doing but aren't; this puts up thick walls that are next to impenetrable.

Like attracts like...It is as simple as that. If you are walking the streets mumbling to yourself how unworthy and worthless you are what do you think you are going to attract? This is even a biblical principle for those of you who think I am just talking mumbo jumbo. This is a book for everyone because new age and Christians alike have Lyme Disease. So many who have this lose faith in everything, as I have struggled with it too. One thing I have found out and strictly believe is a closed mind will not heal one from

Lyme. It's a very complex and voracious disease that you need to treat with all modalities…incorporating absolutely anything and everything to survive this. I also mention auras and chakras in this section, and have supportive biblical scripture to support this. New Agers say we are God, Christians say God made us in his image. It is the same thing, just different verbiage.

Proverbs 15:15 All the days of the afflicted are evil, but he who is of a merry heart has a continual feast. AKJV

What gives you joy? Do you even know? If you do know, and you aren't blessing yourself with it, why?

That's right take out your notebook…

1. I love doing…or you can say for instance "I love spending time with my kids."

Go back to the basics here and doing a page. Again, spend a week or so on this before moving on.

2. Pick three things from your list you love to do or would like to do and do them every day for two weeks. Keep a journal after your joyful duties so you can notice your attitude and how good it feels to be doing those things. You may be surprised at the response you get. People may say to you "Wow, did you do something with your hair?" They won't be able to place what is different and you will not have done your hair…They will be acting in direct response to your joy from completing your joyful duty to yourself.

Step 2. Keeping yourself in check. Below are some exercises to help you on your way to living joy each day.

Breathing Exercise: (This is the precursor to doing the the "yogaesque" exercise (mentioned later.)

WARNINGDo not attempt the breathing exercise while driving. It is extremely relaxing and might make you fall asleep at the wheel.***

(Breathing from your diaphragm) ... If you have a hard time with this place your hand on your stomach and practice breathing until your stomach is pushing on your hand with your breath.

Breathe slow, deep, and steady, in nose to the count of 5 (or what is comfortable for you).

Hold for the count of 5 (or what is comfortable for you).

Exhale out the mouth for the count of 5 (breathing from diaphragm).

(this releases any negative energy that is pent up).

Repeat 5 times or until you feel as if there is a soft breeze around you.

Breathe slow, deep, and steady, in nose to the count of 5 (or what is comfortable for you).

Hold for the count of 5 (or what is comfortable for you).

Exhale out the nose for the count of 5 (breathing from diaphragm).

Repeat 5 times period.

REPEAT CYCLE 3 TIMES.

Now say with conviction either out loud or internally.

I now take back my power and reclaim my authentic self! I am whole I am beautiful…I am at peace, and one with God.

Meditate on that and really feel that power coming back to your center above your navel.

HERE IS WHERE I START TALKING ABOUT AURAS AND CHAKRAS

Go to the next page so this is easier to read and doesn't split the text.

When speaking of chakras, it is said there are seven of them. They are "lights" within ourselves and do spin and flash light and energy. So, keep this in mind as you read this.

Revelation 4:5 Out from the throne come flashes of lightning and sounds and peals of thunder. And there were seven lamps of fire burning before the throne, which are the seven Spirits of God;

NASB

The aura is the ring of rainbowed energy that encapsulates our soul. It is a protective sort of bubble to help protect our soul and even body.

And He who was sitting was like a jasper stone and a sardius in appearance; and there was a rainbow around the throne, like an emerald in appearance.

Revelation 4:3 NASB

So, I think you can see the relation. Continue to try to keep an open mind. The one thing I will say, is that in my opinion; many spirituals out there make things too hard and it isn't. It is as easy as speaking it. The problem is we are human and sometimes we need extra help to calm us down and center like breathing or music even, before we can meditate or heal.

Speak aloud or internally…

1. My aura is limitless!

(Repeat until you have an "expanded" feeling. You will have this feeling I promise. Just keep repeating it.) It might feel like a cool breeze is blowing around you when there isn't any breeze present. It is a very real and living thing.

3. My chakras are completely balanced. (Repeat until you feel the seven centers moving or spinning.

These are:

    a. 1. Between our thighs-Grounding

    b. 2. At our pubic line-Relationships and sexuality

    c. 3. Right above the navel-Our power center

    d. 4. Heart-Love…clearly

    e. 5. Throat-Communication

    f. 6. Brow-Wisdom, and decision making

    g. 7. Top of the head-Connection, inner and outer beauty

Now we are going to activate the God Center located above the heart and below the throat right below that little dip at the bottom of your neck. What is the God Center you may ask? It is where the connection to God and you become solid and whole, and no longer separated. It essentially puts out the life line to you and God. It is a most awesome place of existence to be in. I will tell you however, that there may be some crying not really of sadness but for such divine exhilaration being home with Father/Source/or Universe.

My God center is now activated. (Repeat until you feel that center of your upper chest expanding. Trust me you'll feel it. Prepare yourself to be amazed!)

You will not have to activate this again. The next time you go through these steps, you will simply say "My God center is limitless". (Repeat until you feel the expansion. It will continue on by itself).

Now we are going to start matching our energies to God's. God made us in his own image remember? So, let's step up to the plate.

Our aura has a sort of vibratory motion to it. One that you will be able to feel if you keep your mind open and keep out of your own thought.

My vibration is that of God's. (Repeat until you feel the gentle vibration feeling as if it is going through your veins). Move on to the next page for Step 3.

Step 3. Finding and Embracing Your Center

Once you have done the above steps you will be ready to become centered. This is different than finding your God center. Whereas the above steps are for upkeep, on a daily basis; this is more for meditating and feeling that "enlightened" feeling.

Closing your eyes, hold your arm and hand straight out. Feel the area around you. It will feel a bit cool and maybe breezy. Now draw your hand in right outside of your body. Notice the warmth?

Slowly put your hand down in a resting position.

Draw your attention inward till you find what I call the warm goo phase. This is at the center of your being as in the God center but is more like a thick soft core...think jelly roll, this being the jelly. The more time you spend here the warmer you will feel. It is good to spend about 15 minutes here in this space every day. It can be whenever you wish.

Chapter 4 Taking A Break and Gaining Knowledge

What You May or May Not Know About Lyme

Before I even start in this section, what worked for me might not work for you, or it might. I am not a doctor. I can only speak from my own experience and what helped me. I am not saying you should try what I have out of desperation, I am only sharing with you my journey with this and the things that I have learned so far. I am far from an expert, but perhaps there might be some things here you hadn't thought about.

When I first started getting sick no one knew what was wrong with me. This is the key phrase, as Lyme is considered the great masquerader. The doctors thought this and that were wrong with me. That I had cancer, MS, that it was menopause and gave me a hysterectomy, and a myriad of other things. They did this and that and while I felt better for a short time, it all went back to the same old thing and many times got worse. This is when everyone starts thinking it is all in your head and that you are a hypochondriac…and let me tell you right now there is nothing worse than feeling so incredibly ill and no one believing you, just thinking you are crazy.

Whether you have already been diagnosed or whether you are just venturing out there thinking you have Lyme…

YOU AREN'T CRAZY!!!

Tests don't always register numbers with this. My first Lyme test they claimed was negative. It wasn't; it was in the median zone with the IGM Quantitation and It was my gynecologist who finally gave me my first round of antibiotics. I was persistent with the doctors in the clinic and they didn't like it. If you are not getting anywhere with the doctors, stick up for yourself and be a squeaky wheel even if you have to; practically stage a protest.

What I have gone through I wouldn't wish on my worst enemy even my ex-husband.

If you suspect at all you have Lyme and you aren't getting anywhere start something anything to help yourself at least in the natural department. Look at all the suggestions here in the book and other places and get started on something…anything to see if it will help and at least keep it from getting into something bad such as vital organs.

If you were start at just one place, I would start a gentle detox because Lyme does poison your body. Then slowly start adding things one by one until you notice a light bulb going off …" That's my thing"! I am going to start a list on the next page of the easiest things to acquire with both tried and untried. I do wish somebody would have told me to take a probiotic including the doctors. No one did. When you are in a terrible sick state, your brain doesn't work good enough to think for yourself. I am not scientific really in this book and that is why. I had a terrible time understanding it all and could have used a guide that had it all as A, B, C, D. This is what I have tried to do for you.

What I Have Tried and My Bodies Response to Them in Order

Keep in mind, these are my individual responses. I am very, very, very, sensitive to meds, foods, and the like. Don't let this scare you. Some of these might work for you and for many they do. Just keep in mind if your body is very sensitive or allergic to things I would be very wary.

* Doxycycline Mono 100-(L-form and Spirochete, not safe for children or pregnant women.)This was a total fucking disaster the first time! I started feeling my brain burning right away within a couple of hours. This went on for a for two days and everyone told me this was normal. It wasn't. A Herxheimer response is normal however, not the strange burning I had and "shock' type sensations going on in my brain that felt like a misfire. "Herxing" sucks. This was a hundred times worse. I kept taking it because everyone told me this was normal. I woke up the following morning unable to talk. Every single syllable was stuttered and I mean bad! I had to write out everything. Then I couldn't get the doctors to take me off of it telling me this is the one recommended and I just had to finish it. By the end of the third day I

could barely walk. This also made me text my boyfriend well over forty times in a row. Huge impulse control problems that had been significantly worse than before. I finally had someone make some phone calls to get a referral immediately to a neurologist who told me absolutely; no more! However, he didn't give me anything to follow up on except Gabapentin which helped for about a week. I had to get it upped more and more. No one would help me. I was stuck with a stupid tongue that wouldn't work and grabbing on to the walls in my house for dear life afraid I was going to fall. I could barely get myself off the toilet or out of bed. This lasted two months. Later, I was put back on it to have the same issues.

❖ Clindamycin-(babesiosis found out later should have been with quinine, yet with the two can be risks and is only recommended in mild to moderate cases.) Two months later. Yes, two months it took for someone to help me finally. An on-call doctor who knew of Lyme and that it was clearly in my brain and gave me this one. It did seem to start helping me about the 7-day mark. I improved little by little over a span of about 2 1/2 months. Then that doctor left and I wasn't told and I ran out. I was once again without meds and was still clearly not cured. Due to the fact I had been on it 2 1/2 months doctors told me that was enough and wouldn't even bother testing me again. I was a bit better and some speech returned approximately 30% but was still really stuttering and walking hadn't really improved at all. I think one of the only reasons I felt any better was maybe I caught a co-infection and it got rid of the co-infection.

❖ Other Protocols-This is when I started the mad dog search online for answers, help, and support…and got none. I was having a very hard time finding anything lucrative online. At this point I am going to tell you I am a medium whether it is something you choose you want to believe or not. Let me tell you though, without the help of "M" I wouldn't be sitting here today or functioning at all without her help. She would go and gather information and keywords for me to type in to find these other things to try. Remember, I had no support of family really, live in a remote area, and was having a serious brain issue that made it very hard for me to do anything with searches. Just continue to keep an open mind as you keep reading about this journey "M" helped me with.

- ❖ Vitamin C/Salt Protocol-(Nothing substantial out there on what forms) I am very sensitive to salt and decided that wouldn't work those combinations to we had to find something else to go with it somehow. I did however start taking mega-doses of Vit C alone starting at 5,000 mg a day, going up to 50,000 mg daily. There is Vitamin C body tolerance to pay close attention to. You know how sick you are and how much you need by what your body does. If you have a high tolerance for it without loose stools; you know how sick you are. You will have very, very, loose stools if you take too much, but just take a little less and that will go away. If this happens drop it down by 1,000 mg at a time. Our bodies do not produce Vitamin C on its' own so supplementation for many of us is necessary. After about a week of this which is pretty good timing, I started feeling better just on this and some speech returned and I was walking better. I didn't seem to have much "herxing" at all from this and at least I was upright and out of bed. I think this helped primarily because it boosted my immune system to try to fight them naturally. I still believe in this as an addition but not a sole option. I still needed extra help.

- ❖ Claritin or Loratadine-(prevents manganese absorption to the bacteria and does seem to kill some. The problem is there is not enough known as to the safety to the human body and I am only giving you my information on my individual choice to use it.) I found this little miracle in a study "she" led me to at Stanford University that had just come out within the last 30 days at this point. If given in-vitro at 400x the dose LOL it was found to kill the spirochete. Clearly, I couldn't take 400x, but I was already taking 2 at a time for allergies that seemed to get worse since contracting Lyme. So, slowly I started upping the Claritin (which I got at Costco, Kirkland brand). I took two in the morning and two in the evening and I did notice a little more difference but not enough. After a few more days I took 4 in the morning and 4 in the evening. It did make me nauseated, but it also made me function better. Little by little my body adapted to the amount I was taking and slowly I was improving with little "herxing". I drank detox tea I will list later and seemed to be holding my own for a while and kept improving. I even started walking again and doing some belly dancing. I was concerned though It wasn't doing the job and couldn't get anyone to retest me or give me any other antibiotic. Then as all good things must end, I was having issues again. This could have been from neurotoxins from the spirochetes releasing their stinking, farting, gas inside of me. I wasn't sure exactly how to get rid of them. So, then she led me to…

- ❖ Infra-red Saunas-(Extreme heat will kill spirochetes.) Ohhhh, it felt so beautifully relaxing and I slept all night. However, the next day…holy shit! It was terrible. No one had stated anywhere that you needed to take a good shower afterwards to get the toxins off your skin or they soak back in and can make you sicker and give you horrible rashes and sores. I felt so ill and was in bed for weeks before the effects of it finally tapered off. I didn't like it Sam I am. BIG, BIG, NO BUENO!!! NO!!! I continued on with the Vitamin C and Claritin for 2 months. Then we found…

- ❖ Grape Fruit Seed Extract (cyst), Cinnamon Oil (antimicrobial, borrelia), Wild Mountain Oregano (it is said this kills all forms when taken at the right dose. So ask your naturopath.) and Stevia (all forms). All of these will also kill probiotics if taken at same time so take ProB at least two hours later)-I was actually amazed. I went through some pretty serious "herxing" but nothing I couldn't handle and I wasn't "herxing" all the time. I still wasn't back to normal after this though so things were added in seeing things posted by others, and were adding just as much if not more to their own protocol.

Then it hit! Again! With the impulse control it was terrible! My poor boyfriend got texted I don't know how many times! I was going to lose this man if something wasn't done. I knew he was trying to understand but I was a neurotic mess and had been for a fucking year, on and off. I couldn't stand myself…this illness anymore and I couldn't lose the most important, pivotal, person in my life. I finally passed out from exhaustion thank gawd but not until I had already been blowing up his fucking phone for probably 3-4 hours! When I think about it all now when I am semi-normal, I am so hmm…humiliated…and crying. The man is a saint. It makes me very, very, sad to think he doesn't even know who I really am, because of this fucking, bullshit, mother fucking, disease.

I woke the next morning, and oh my fucking gawd the pain! It was indescribable! I had been in a lot of pain but I have a high pain tolerance and had been holding my own. I couldn't talk again and found out when at the hospital in a different city 30 min. away I couldn't write my name either to sign papers. It was humiliating. I didn't know how to spell my name and had to look at my license then figured out I couldn't write hardly at all. Finally, registered for the ER I sat and waited for three hours before deciding to leave and go to another hospital.

Reluctantly and with fight they hospitalized me and gave me Doxy 100 IV and had me hopped up on pain meds. No interaction like before and within 4 days I was feeling better…thank you pain meds. There were doctors there on the floor though that did not like that I was there. They gave me a horrid time because there was no "proof". A doctor who apparently hadn't had enough sex or something comes in like a banshee and discharges me no IV because a test came back negative for the Western Blot. That was it. I cried and cried and was completely inconsolable. Then in a last moment of clarity as I left I grabbed the IV bag and walked out with it. LOL So I could maybe show another doctor and since I was doing better on it maybe I could talk them into it. So, I called my local clinic that day right before closing time. Got an appointment for about 4 days later. Finally, another "traveling doctor" was covering at the clinic.

❖ Minocycline (Bb, cyst, neuroborreliosis, penetrates cell walls, ok for pregnancy but can permanently stain the teeth of the baby in utero, and of children also, not recommended for children under 8) I was in so much pain, crying and shaking and begging her to help me. She was beautifully sensitive to my needs. She knew of Lyme well, and gave me Minocycline orally. I had issues that same night with chest pain and head thought I was having a heart attack or stroke. She said that's it with that and put me in the hospital on Doxy 100 IV which I agreed to since I would have some supervision. I was done and desperate. She however was only there for a few weeks when I found her. She wanted me admitted for three weeks.

I was elated! Then I find out when she admits me she was leaving in two days and another doctor was going to be there. I was doing better and speech very slowly improving not writing so much or walking. The doctor seemed nice enough who was taking over for her but something made me feel uneasy. With a week left to my treatment the covering doctor got a bee up his ass and got in a fight with her about my being there longer. I was discharged without her approval. Immediately I made an appointment, to what would be my last appointment with her upon her return.

When she came back with two days left to her work stint at the clinic, it already wasn't a good day. I was in horrific pain, my mom wouldn't give me a ride, and while my son said he'd take me he begrudgingly did it. I went in knowing she was going to do standard blood work on me. She comes in with an odd look on her face. Sits down. looks at me with tears in her eyes. "I think it's time to test you for malignancies." We have done everything and you just aren't healing." I took a breath and sat there. I had

wondered myself. I sighed. I asked her how many malignancies there were that were

possibilities with my symptoms. She told me five. She gave me the order paper,

embraced me, told me it was going to be okay, and that was it. Three hours later. My son

yelled at me so bad; people turned around in the parking lot. I was trying to keep it to

myself and just lost it. "Stop yelling at me!!! She's testing me for cancers!" I wept and

wept. He takes off like a bat out of hell, pulls over and says "Mom, that's a dick fucking

move.!" I told him to not talk to me and take me home. Test results were supposed to be

within two days. It took a week.

I called and called the clinic and no one would give me the results of the tests. I mean

no one. I was her patient so they wouldn't give them to me and they had to call her they

said. So I waited…and waited. Then they tell me they couldn't get hold of her.

So, I go home and start looking for her. It took me three days. I found her on a social

network site. She being the kind person she was, told me the answer. Positive cancer

protein for neuroendocrine, bone, and thyroid. My heart sank. She said the numbers were low indicating in early stages which was good. It could be nothing, and maybe even related to Lyme. She didn't think so though.

I told a few members of my family and my boyfriend. Of course, he was supportive.

I continued to talk to this doctor here and there. Still having issues and in so much pain and crying uncontrollably. "M" tells me to type in to Google antibiotics to kill early stages of cancer. I thought I was surely losing my mind, I did it though; because she's never wrong. Sure, enough it was there. Not only was it there but the one that had the best report so far was Minocycline. I messaged the doctor right away and she said she said she had seen that. I still had Minocycline left and started taking it but I was going to run out. I did however have refills. So, she called in to my pharmacy and gave me all these refills and told me to not go off them for six months.

I knew I had issues before but I was desperate but it was better than losing my hair if I indeed had it and maybe it would kill two birds with one stone. I could relax a little and not have to fight with doctors. Maybe would help my body rest.

As is with this disease always, I started having problems with it and it got worse and worse. This is where I went off the antibiotics I spoke of earlier because I was afraid of damage to my brain, and here I sit. Still no other doctor or help or knowing if I have cancer or if it is Lyme causing those reads which is possible; to get a false cancer read. This had happened two time before already with thyroid and something else I can't even remember. Then I was fine. I'm trying to trust I am. It is hard.

So now I wait for this other doctor. Let the games begin!

❖ IGF-1(Hormone balancing: dealing with the thyroid, reproductive, adrenals, pituitary, energy enhancing, reducing thick blood and clotting (a common in Lyme), anti-inflammatory, immune function, increased strength in nerves and muscles just to name a few) However, I will mention this first: There is argument out there that this has been linked to some cancers.

I guess my thing on this is, the medical community is always changing their mind with something. It's good for us, it isn't, and back and forth with it. Just like how you should put babies on their belly to sleep. It has changed about ten times in the last twenty years and gone back and forth what you should do. I will also say though, there is enough question at hand about the honesty of the FDA and pharmaceutical companies when we are dealing with supplements. I do not question at all the validity, and helpfulness of medications in the market. I just feel however there needs to be a broader outlook in possibly combining the usefulness of both.

What I do know, is I feel better on it. I have cancer in my family. So, who knows why I tested positive. I could have also tested positive from the stupid Lyme bacteria also. They have found a relation to cancer and Lyme patients as well.

Here is where it gets interesting. There have also been studies showing IGF-1 eradicates cancer. So, which is true?

I know it has helped me so this is why; I have gone back to taking it and will be continuing. I personally like the one I bought. There are many. I will be leaving the name of it under resources in this book. I also suggest using muscle testing which I will be going into at greater length in its own section.

As with everything. If there is a question, do your own research. Get your IGM levels tested. I have not yet because all the doctors down here have been idiots except one and I didn't know about the IGM-1 then. This book is just about giving you a guide to read and access so on the days you feel like shit, and the world is ending, on the days you just can't sit up on the net or look at your phone one more time. You have this. It is just to help educate you, on things you might not know, and an intimate look into someone like you who has tried to make sense out of it all without all the scientific language that can be daunting and confusing, especially to someone who has Lyme in the brain.

* Tru-Light Therapy by Mellen Thomas-(Calming and soothing to the nerves, purifies the blood(shortened definition)-During one of the times I was at my worst and really struggling ready to give up, I was talking to my mom about the Bob Beck Magnetic

Pulser and that it went on the wrist and was supposed to purify the blood. I

mentioned I didn't however like the thought of little shocks (compared to that of a

TENS unit). She had a funny look on her face…she left…she comes back with this

device. She said it wasn't the one she had, that she had purchased it back in the

1980s. There is a lot of information out there and some are very skeptical. I will tell

you though, this machine was making a difference for me. You are supposed to put it

on your wrist where your two main veins are or other part of the body but head

hadn't been mentioned. It had a strap to wrap it around and secure so you didn't have

to hold it. I put it anywhere I could. When I put it on my head I put on my temple

areas for about 15 min each. I could feel something moving around in my brain but it

was a soothing movement, healing, as opposed to something eating my brain. It

helped me sleep, and I found it very helpful to just help me be peaceful. As to the

medical proof…I am not sure about that; but I loved it. It made me at least 70% more

comfortable and at least took the edge off.

I have looked on the internet for these and I can't find anything. I will list the

company in resources and they might be able to lead you to one. He has a new device out

now I cannot speak for, but there does seem to be a following. You can view some videos by doing a search on YOUTUBE and at your own conclusion. I do feel however it is

worth exploring.

* ❖ Chaga Mushroom Tea-(immune boosting, nerves and stress, energy, inflammation,

  oxygen boosting to cells) I love Chaga. You can find it ground and while most

  people made a tea with it I ate it LOL. Tastes a bit like chicory. Highly

  recommended.

* ❖ Stevia-(B. burgdorferi spirochetes, persister forms, and many others. Compared to be

  as effective if not more than antibiotics in studies) I have found Stevia helps to keep

  me sane as well during the die off, and deal with neurotoxins as opposed to when I

  don't take it. That however is my own experience. It is single handedly the one thing

  that killed my Lyme. I took Now brand 8 oz. bottle 1 tsp. 4 times a day until gone.

* ❖ Garlic Pills-(soft gel over 1,000 mg, antimicrobial, natural antibiotic, and protects

  against co-infections)

- ❖ Curry Powder-As a cheaper alternative to turmeric which without pepper does nothing. Check labels with curry powder to make sure no MSG is in there and that it has pepper. I am actually a curry whore. LOL I put it on everything! Avocadoes, eggs…everything! During a time that I was at my worst, I used to run hot water through my Keurig and have a mug of curry broth. It was very soothing. About a tsp. or so at a time. Drank it all day.

- ❖ Cannabis-The form I tried was in butter. I only took 3 oz of butter and wasn't regular with it. I didn't like how I felt on it. It did however help me sleep unlike anything else. I was probably having issues with the "herxing" that did happen after taking it. It just wasn't for me, but doesn't mean it wouldn't work for you. The oil form I have heard others rave about including the Rick Simpson Oil. If this nonsense continues I might be going back to this. As for right now it is not for me.

- ❖ Vicks Vapor Rub-Yup, Vicks. I used the cheapo stuff. It helped my pain, itching, and I put it on my feet to help draw out toxins gently which seemed to help. It was very calming an soothing during "herxing". I am still using it sometimes like a "blanky".

To smell it calms my brain quite a bit.

- ❖ Boswellia-I didn't find out about Boswellia until after. I was having a lot of issues

  with chronic brain inflammation and pain still that sometimes was just too much for

  me. It is the ticket for me to leading a half-way normal life now. I wish I would have

  known about it during the "heat" of my illness.

- ❖ Coconut Oil, Organic-This is what I feel protected my brain. I still take it every day

  to hopefully get some of my brain back. Build up with it though a teaspoon at a time

  until you are at a TBS. a day.

- ❖ Listening To Geto Boys~Die Mother Fucker (based on Messages From Water by Dr.

  Emoto) I will tell you this much…There is something to this because I have felt my

  most intense "herxing" from listening to this song. Yet, it seems to put me in a better

  mood and balances me amazingly…perhaps because my Lyme…(lol "my Lyme") is

  in my brain and nervous system. More about this later.

Other Drug, Supplement, And Misc. Protocols I Haven't Tried

➢ Bob Beck Magnetic Pulser- Purifies Blood

➢ Rife Machine-Electronic Along the Same Lines

➢ The Milk Cure

➢ Allicin-(I realized later, much later in my own treatment protocol that I had been taking it. Garlic powder. It's cheaper than Allicin and has a higher Allicin content.

➢ Bee Venom

The Following Are Just Lists Of Antibiotics and Natural Remedies Used For Treatment Of Lyme-(you can ask your physician about them). If you treat naturally, DO NOT take all of these all at once! A few at a time after doing some research to see how they mix well together. If you are taking antibiotics ask your pharmacist about known reactions with any herbal remedy you use, and of course muscle test.

For Cystic Form:

> Spheroplast or Cell Wall Deficient-Plaquenil

> Grapefruit Seed Extract

> Tindamax

> Flagyl

Biofilms:

> Lauricidin

> Stevia-This is what eventually killed my Lyme.

> Serrapeptase

> Nattokinase

> Raw Garlic

> Curcumin

> Turmeric

- ➤ Lactoferrin

- ➤ Bladderwrack

- ➤ Xylitol

- ➤ Guaifenesin Maximum-Strength Mucinex (I actually took some being sick one time. OH MY GAWD! I nearly went off the deep end. It is said People with Lyme shouldn't take it because it can cause MAJOR "herxing"…UM YEAH! Now as I think about it, perhaps it kills more than biofilms. I felt like shit! I am kind of afraid to try it myself again, that is how bad it was. Reconsidering now though. I don't know I would do this one. It was bad.

- ➤ Sarsaparilla

- ➤ Extra Virgin Coconut Oil (I have just started using this specifically by TBS now to help put my brain back together after finding out about studies shown to be beneficial for Alzheimer's.

- ➤ Neem Oil

- ➤ Boswellia for brain inflammation, thinning blood (a problem for "Lymies" thick blood) relief from anxiety, depression, and chronic pain. It has been a miracle for me.

For Intracellular Form:

➢ Rifampin

➢ Macrolides (azithromycin, clarithromycin, roxithromycin,)

➢ Quinolones (ciprofloxicin, levaquin, avelox, factive)

➢ Gentamicin

➢ Dapsone

➢ Tetracyclines (Monocycline, tetracycline HCL, doxycycline)

➢ Pyrazinamide

For Cell Form:

➢ Vancomycin

➢ Primaxin

➢ Suprax

➢ Omnicef

- ➢ Bicillin

- ➢ Claforan

- ➢ Rocephin

- ➢ Augmentin

- ➢ Cedax

- ➢ Amoxicillin

These lists are just meant to get you started. I have picked the main, and basic one's for you that are the easiest to attain, and that I have personally used for other reasons. Please use caution in taking any of these and use your own judgment above all and listen to that inner-voice.

Muscle Testing to Find Out What Will Fit Your Body

This will probably be the shortest section of this book but one of the most valuable.

I have used muscle testing for over twenty years for everything from allergies, foods, supplements, medications, for myself and my children. The process is different for yourself than when you test on others. You can use this for anything to find out what will be a good fit for your body. Just like anything else out there in the metaphysical area, people like to try to make too much out of this. I am going to make this very easy for you.

Sit in a chair or up in your bed. Put the item you are wondering about in your lap or on you anywhere. Even in your bra. Get the item let's say, "coffee" in your mind. Take your thumb and middle finger of both hands and link them together. Quiet your mind. Now ask is this good for my body? Really concentrate on the question. Make sure your fingers are as tight as you can hold. Now try to pull your fingers apart. If the link comes apart or is weak it is not good for you. If you can't pull apart or it's hard, it's okay. Easy.

Want to do it on other people? Or have others do it to you? Stand or sit with the strongest arm straight out, to the side of you is best. Hold the item with your opposite hand (strong, dominant, arm) and concentrate on it then have them try to push the arm down while resisting. If the arms goes down easy it's a no. If can't really push down on it it's a yes.

You can use the same processes to find out if an activity would wear you out too much or going to the store just by thinking it. Including certain doctors. Your body subconsciously knows what's right for it. Think, link, pull. Easy.

So, for example, let's say you go to the store alone. You want to know if a cereal is okay for you. Look at it. Focus on it. Think, link, and pull. That's all there is to it.

I have used this as well for traveling to make sure a trip would be safe for travel. Only to find out many times over there were fatal accidents on the day I would have traveled. Same process. Think, link, and pull.

Have fun with it and even get your children or grandchildren involved. I used to do this with my kids. My kids used to play games with it to tease their siblings. "I just asked my fingers if you should have that and they said no". LOL "Nuh uh…prove it". They'd take like a candy bar in one hand. Sibling push on the other. "Oh, man!".

You can use this for your pets too. Just by focusing your mind. Think, (Should Spot have this treat?) link, pull. :-)

Here is what I have to say about this. There is so much info out there, it's mind numbing, and especially if it is in the brain or you have this "brain fog". Just like with anything else a person can really drive themselves crazy with it. Educate yourself yes but don't drive yourself crazy. I believe in making things easy. We have a hard enough job healing our body and keeping sane; without these huge long lists and what to do and not do. I have had quite a few co-infections myself, including the swine flu. This would not have happened I am sure if I had been taking Vitamin C as well as garlic pills or Allicin. They will not interfere with antibiotics and help keep your immune system functioning. How much depends on your body. So, listen to it. Your body is smart. Do muscle testing to find out your dosage.

While raw garlic is fine if you must eat it to ward off vampires LOL, I would stick to putting it in dishes because it can tear up your stomach if in large doses and even cause bleeding in the stomach and intestines. Trust me.

Unfortunately, we have become a society that banks on impressing fear on us for their own gain. I am not about that. Listen to yourself and arrive at your own conclusions. Doctors while they know some things aren't God and do not know everything. I have been told I'd never have kids…had five, that I had cancer and wasn't pregnant when I was and didn't have cancer, that I would always have a heart condition which I don't, that my daughter would never run or jump again as a result of a terrible break, above all that I didn't have Lyme and I did…and this isn't all of it.

Please, please, please, if you got nothing more from this book than this…I would be happy. Please; listen to your own "inner voice". Not mine or anyone elses. Yours. Our subconscious mind knows our body (more on that later). We were programmed that way. This is the main purpose of this book really, educate lightly, teach you of your inner voice so you can heal yourself more effectively, and make you laugh from my undying, wit and raw humor.

Yes, co-infections are a huge problem for Lymies. However, just use common sense. Take Vitamin C, garlic whatever mode, DO NOT overexert yourself, and carry disinfectant wipes with you and hand sanitizer when you go to the stores and wipe things before you touch them. Including the nasty pin pads at the stores, even if people give you

nasty looks and roll their eyes…and use hand sanitizer.

❖ Pregnancy and Breastfeeding:

Someone requested a section on pregnancy and breastfeeding. Listen, pregnancy is supposed to be a beautiful experience. Treat it as such. The above follows for this. Can Lyme affect the fetus? Yes. Can it get into the breast milk? Yes. It can. Does it mean they will no. For every handful of women who have had miscarriages, or stillborn, birth defects…supposedly from Lyme, there's a handful of women who haven't.

Talk to your doctor. Make sure you are taking a safe antibiotic for pregnancy. Vitamin C and Garlic are both safe for pregnancy (to go with the antibiotic not alone). I took them the whole time with all 5 because of my asthma.

As far as your breast milk? Breast milk has macrophages that eat up germs and protects against infection and disease. I know this because I took breastfeeding classes to work as a Breastfeeding Peer Counselor. If you are concerned about it you can have your breast milk tested for the Lyme bacteria to be safe.

It can be passed to the baby yes. My oldest was recently tested by my forcing him to

do so. It showed he had the antibody, but there was nothing else. He is 29, and drives me

nuts! So far there is nothing else with my kids. I breastfed all of them, and two of them at

the same time until they were 3 and 4 years old. No, they weren't twins.

❖ Infertility:

Lyme can get into the uterus and cause some problems and in the ovaries as well, and with hormones. However, it is not impossible. There are simple things you can do to help this without going through a whole lot to start.

➢ 3 months prior to trying to get pregnant, take orally or drink Damiana tea, as well as wild yam root. Find organic progesterone cream at the health food store to help balance you out, and take Folic Acid 800 mg.

➢ Test Your Iron and Iron Stores-This means not just hemoglobin. Make them check your Ferritin which are your iron stores. If you are anemic you will not ovulate correctly or produce healthy swimmers.

➢ NO CAFFEINE! NONE. Or smoking including pot.

➢ Keep his "boys" cool on ice, you hot. Perhaps even use a heating pad over your lower belly.

➢ Intercourse every 48 hours. Not daily and only once.

➢ Get on your hands and knees and put your head down. After he ejaculates, stay there for at least 20 minutes. Then carefully roll over and on your back, and put a pillow under your rear just for slight elevation. Anything other that, could block the flow.

➢ Don't always plan it. Men hate that. Get him excited and worked up instead. Men are primal naughty beasts…and let's face it we love them that way. Try sending him maybe sexy texts, or emails, or even sexy phone calls, and going as far to talk very dirty. Make it sexy for him. Tell him what a glorious beast he is. Tell him all the dirty things you want to do to him and how much he pleases your body. Don't just make it about having a baby. He counts too, and he needs to know that. You know your man. You know what he himself as an individual likes. However, men will also to avoid consternation…tend just do what he thinks will make his woman happy which is fine, but will also lower his sperm count.

To get those fishies swimming; get his boys hot, and tease the bone. Work up the day before and not to completion.

Above all, have fun making a baby. Don't make it a chore. Choose to make it memorable instead.

The chance of sexual transmission on the next page.

Sexual Transmission?

Just like with the above info with pregnancy and breastfeeding and transferring to the fetus or baby, there are varied opinions on this subject. I will tell you I have seen more articles that it isn't sexually transmitted than it is. The best article I have found so far is from:

https://www.aldf.com/pdf/Letter_to_the_editor_of_AFMR_for_ALDF_website_3.10.14.pdf.

This is why, I tell you not to be fearful or believe everything you read. This is just meant as a guide and you have to arrive at your own conclusions. No one person, doctor, or scientist knows everything. We are all human. There is however, enough info out there speaking about transmission to fetus, baby, or sexually…that over and over it is just not something to become overly fearful about so that it ruins your life. Ya' know? Again, for every handful of people that there "seems" to be a connective tissue with this as far as transmission, there is a handful out there with no link.

From the research I have done it is in my opinion saying it is transferred by the above means would be like saying if you were to have cancer: by having sex with my woman or man they'd get cancer, or my baby would get cancer. The results are unfounded.

Our fight is hard enough without the predisposed fear put on us by media etc. Just educate yourselves and be at peace.

- In public places and bathrooms wipe down before you touch, sit, flush, or wash.

- WIPE DOWN THOSE CARTS!!!! ON ALL EDGES ETC.

- At a meat counter or handling even packaged meat, carry disposable gloves with you.

- STAY AWAY FROM SAND BOXES!

- Watch cleaning litter boxes.

- Watch public pools, saunas, hot tubs, massage tables (make sure you see them wipe it down) lakes and gyms.

- If you wish to exercise, seriously just get DVDs until you are better. Just try to walk if you can. Stay away from the gyms. They are bacteria breeders.

- Schools and Institutions-Follow the above rules. Use good sense and just educate your kids. Whether its to prevent them bringing something home to mom and dad or to protect your Lil' Lymie.

- Have your floors cleaned regularly, and leave shoes outside.

✧ Wipe down Fido's feet if indoor dog with baby wipes. It only takes a minute. Even better to get those cute little doggie shoes.

✧ Keep cats inside.

✧ Wipe your mail down.

You get the picture. This is just until your immune system is stronger and you have been on Vitamin C and garlic for a while.

Symptoms Lyme Disease

I have tried to compile a very complete list on all the varying symptoms of Lyme. Some might be familiar some might not be. Please use your own discretion when assessing your symptoms. Realize these might come and go and typically do; and do not stop sitting on doctors just because they keep telling you there's nothing wrong with you. Stay on them. It's your health on the line and possibly your life. It is your right. In addition, you may find a Lyme checklist to download here http://www.lymeresearchalliance.org/PDF/signs/lyme-disease-checklist.pdf.

- You are sicker than hell for no known reason, in and out of hospitals, doctor's office for varying reasons and they can't figure out what's wrong with you.

- Sudden mood swings, sometimes so intense can make you appear bipolar or psychotic when no previous history has been prevalent.

- Obsessiveness sudden OCD

- Insomnia

- Facial paralysis

- Optic Neuritis

- Constant fatigue

- Neck pressure, pain, and creaking or cracking of the neck

- Dental issues and pain

- Burning, shooting pain, stabbing pain, numbness, tingling, hypersensitivity

- Lightheaded, dizzy, off balance, falling a lot, suddenly accident prone, motion sickness, vertigo

- Hearing issues, pain in ears, ringing or buzzing in ears, weepy ears

- Excessive night sleep and or needing to nap a lot during the day

- Vision issues-losing sight, seeing spots, extreme vision changes, eye pain

- Light and sound sensitivity

- Headaches, tremors, seizures

- Feeling the need to be alone to the point of being a recluse

- Anxiety and panic attacks

◆ Speech issues

◆ Confusion, "head fog", things easy before becoming a struggle i.e. (math or spelling)

◆ Short term memory loss

◆ Impulse control issues

◆ Long term memory loss

◆ Sudden weight gain or loss

◆ Disorientation

◆ Forgetfulness

◆ Reading comprehension issues

◆ Muscle pain, twitching, cramps, "charlie horses", anywhere including in the tongue and mouth area

◆ Muscle weakness

◆ Pain or weakness in the back

◆ Spinal pressure

◆ Joint swelling anywhere

◆ Sore feet

◆ Fevers

◆ Persistent swollen glands

◆ Sore throat

◆ Genital, reproductive, and anal pain

◆ Sharp chest and or back pain that might feel like a heart attack

◆ Menstrual issues

◆ Breast pain and or sudden production of milk

◆ Irritable bladder, incontinence issues (including bowels)

◆ Frequent diarrhea

◆ Frequent constipation

◆ Bladder infections and UTI's

◆ Impotence

◆ Loss of libido in men and women

- Sudden overactive and increased sex drive

- Sudden inability to orgasm or difficulty achieving orgasm

- Nausea and frequent motion sickness

- Heartburn and stomach pain

- Persistent pain in the pancreas and liver area

- Persistent intestinal pain

- Sudden uncontrollable vomiting, retching, dry heaves

- Heart issues, irregular heartbeat, palpitations

- Sore ribs

- Irregular EKG

- Chronic cough

- Persistent thick mucus in the throat

- Breathing issues

- Temperature changes

- Night sweats/Sudden chills

- Craving alcohol

- Sudden "addictive" behavior

- Worsened and or exaggerated symptoms after drinking

- Symptoms go away and flare up every few weeks

- Hair loss

- Gaining in body hair in women

- Nail fungus

- Candida that will not go away

- Persistent yeast infections

- Persistent water retention swelling that won't go away

- Brain swelling and sudden Intracranial Hypertension

- Fits of crying and or laughter for no reason

- Presence of H. Pylori while not always or absolute is often a precursor to Lyme Disease

- Halitosis

- Chronic dry throat, itchy throat

- Problems swallowing

- Frequent bruising

- Hypoglycemia even after a meal

- Thick blood (please, please, have your platelets checked)

- Colds and flu that hang on

- Anemic and low iron stores (Ferritin)

- "Cyst" type nodules on body-usually benign

- "Dumping" of nutrients (vitamins and minerals) and chronically riding the low "normal" range, no matter usage of supplements or diet. Your body just can't seem to catch up.

- Inconclusive cancer tests, tests that are positive, then negative, positive and all over the board.

Even if you have just one symptom but it seems to be persistent, stay on your physician about it. Perhaps mention; "Just let me try an antibiotic, if I get better and/or have "herxing" symptoms we know it is probably Lyme. I will not hold you responsible." It is just a thought. I did this. Still, some won't listen to you. Just keep trying.

I personally had most of these issues and without positive tests at first. It is possible to have a multitude of symptoms and nothing to show in tests. This is the problem. Lyme is considered "the great masquerader". You just have to; stay on it.

These are my own personal experiences as well as information I have gathered in speaking with others. Your might have different experiences, or you might have the same. Just because you might only have extreme fatigue doesn't mean you don't have it. Keep exploring and be willing to educate yourself as much as possible and again, don't use this book as your end all be all. Keep exploring your options.

Diet

One word…Pshaw! Here are a couple more…diet, schmiet. Like the earlier

section…Use your own inner voice. Use muscle testing. Yes, it really, really, works. Yes,

it is important to be healthy and eat right in every circumstance. However, just because a

danish bothers you today, doesn't mean it will tomorrow. Then you'll be robing yourself

maybe of the only pleasant thing that day by denying yourself that danish. It would be no

different than saying don't have sex because spreading your legs too long when you have

Lyme might do damage to your joints. Yes, I had someone tell me that. It is ridiculous. I

am sorry if my boyfriend is in front of me he's getting it! LOL. If my body wants a

danish I am eating it, and maybe a damned cookie too, as well as my coffee in the

morning (which we are not supposed to do either). My morning java is almost as good as

having an orgasm in my mouth. Almost.

Me? I tend to live on the edge anyway. I have worried about food intake my entire life

and I am just done with it. If I want a glass or two of wine or a stiff drink, a danish, etc.

I'm gonna do it. Am I going to do it every day? No. Sometimes maybe LOL. As a whole;

I use good sense. As I know you will too.

As important as it is to eat right so our bodies can heal, it is just as important to enjoy ourselves and "be in the presence of lady bugs". Fighting Lyme is tough and debilitating enough without robing yourself of simple, beautiful, yummy, pleasures of all kinds. Use your own discretion and just live your life.

Chapter 5

The Most Important Decision You'll Make~The Decision to Live

Don't you just love "herxing"? Don't you just fucking love it? Yesterday I felt so beat

up. I had been feeling a little better then yesterday it hit me, and hit hard. Then because

the stupid shit is in my brain yada, yada, there's the constant feeling of doom! At times

and you feel like bugs are crawling through your brain and spine and you feel like your

skin is crawling. There is a part of me that just wants to give up...just lay down and say

fuck it come eat me like a fucking buffet. I however, am thinking of this book I started.

That somewhere in the midst of my hell was birthed a little seed...the pull was so great

from somewhere...that someone asked for help...so I don't know who might be helping

who, who might be saving who??? Me and my little imperfect book, or ya' all and

me...giving me, myself hope. That somehow, I might make it out of this fairly unscathed

and alive.

It has been very easy to get lost in this whole God forsaken Lyme thing…in the whole

misery aspect of it.

I think at this stage it is so important especially for those of us who are in what is

considered the "late stages" of Lyme or "chronic", that we get very, very clear with

ourselves, that we are not going to give up! Believe me I know. I know what you all are

going through. As I sit here writing this, I am persecuting myself, calling myself a

hypocrite…because I myself want to just die; if there is no help for me.

I worked so hard to lose my weight and get healthy, for what? To get sick? To lose my

ability to speak, write, type at times, draw, do clay, dance, and do kettlebell? What did I

work so hard for?

If I gave up, I'd be giving up on my kids, my grandkids, future great grandkids…and

that beautiful man of mine; and his beautiful, adorable daughter. Along with any type of

beautiful life we might share together. It is the same for you. Perhaps, you might be someone who thinks they are alone, perhaps no family, no love…and you are sitting there…"Woman just shut the fuck up! You don't know my hell!" "Easy for you to say, I am alone." You are not alone anymore. I am here…and at the end of the book my contact information will be listed for you to reach out to for support. Somehow, I heard your whisper…I felt deep in my heart your feeling of "loneliness" and started writing just for you.

Together, we can change things if we make up our minds, and get clear what we want. We can change the support systems out there (which to be honest aren't great). We can change the insurance companies, the medical system, the legislature…everything.

You really want to allow this to win? There is a reason you felt the need to read this book. In your soul; somewhere, is the will to fight…and I am right there with you fighting as well. I want you to consider just one thing…just one; before you give up. What if darling, there was someone else out there like you? Someone, who like you is at the end of their rope. What if this person got even less help than you? What would you tell them? Consider this…

It has been one hell of a week. I couldn't seem to write or do anything. So, I just sat, laid down, sat some more, drank, slept, in a vicious circle. This is a hard time of year anyway and this makes it even better. I thought the "herxing" would be gentler on the extracts…NOT! It is almost worse. It seems to not be doing anything, then BOOM! Any energy I had built up…gone. When I was on the antibiotics, the last time I just couldn't do it anymore. It caused something so sever in my brain, the horrific pain I was in, stopped overnight. This you might say is great. I however knew this wasn't normal. I mean I felt, nothing. With the help of coconut oil, and taking my supplements listed, I am starting to feel things again…good from a brain standpoint, but from a body standpoint no. I am aware now as I write this; just how bad my body had been hurting all that time, and the pain is coming back. The thought of going through it again is frightening.

The "herxing" this time on the supplements seems to have caused an even worsening depression, and it is all I could even do to write this. This time I am doing it for my boyfriend…so I can make him proud that I just didn't roll over and give up, and somehow something good would come out of this. Now, wouldn't that be a kick in the fucking crotch!

The poor man has really dealt with a lot from me through this. Embarrassingly, so. Perhaps he will be able to see the other sides of me through this. My bad assery, humor, even in bullshit, my beauty; in my loving nature, and that I am quite the fucking "gem". Even among the loss of intelligence, my forgetfulness, the impulse problems, the still occasional stuttering that will probably never go away, the limp that makes me look like I have a corn cob shoved up my ass. That still in there somewhere…is still a semi-graceful, beautiful, loving, gifted, woman…who is worth hanging onto, touching, loving, loving, loving…and touching some more. I just need a day of rest and fun…where instead of feeling like I have bugs crawling over me and up my ass to the point I want to play dog and scoot along the fucking carpet all the time (who knows if it's because I am still infected or just brain damage from what lurked there before). So that I feel him touching me, caressing me, grabbing me…making me feel like a woman again…instead of a bad cartoon…like only he can do. Now, I know my happiness can't come from him. This…however, is a shit fucking ass disease that has kicked my ass and I deserve some TLC and beyond God damnit…way, way, way, beyond! Just some time…to forget everything with that beautiful, Portuguese, god; hovering over me.

Since I got really, sick this has been a problem. I always think he is going to leave. It comes from other deep-rooted pain I thought I had dealt with, and because of the loss of brain mass or cells whatever they are…I can't just cope or stuff this fucking shit like I used to. It has done something to my coping mechanism.

Unfortunately, it all seems to be coming out. Sometimes, all at once like a fucking explosion. I am so tired of this cycle like many of you. Where do I go from here? I am still waiting for this stupid doctor appointment, that is like the fucking holy grail. I do not know what I am going to do if they do not help me. This is where this chapter starts coming together and why I chose to write this book. If we are to heal to really heal, we'd better damn well get very, very, clear that's what we want and see out target, aim, shoot as a unified whole…and NEVER FUCKING LOOK THE FUCK BACK!

This, is the sole purpose of this book. To help you on your path to healing. In all things there must be a balance. Medicines, natural remedies, and us getting in touch with our souls…that spiritual side of ourselves that is getting ignored and that is screaming out, trying to get our attention…so we can live. This; is why I have added these exercises for you in this book. To help you deal with the anger, sadness, grief, pain and everything else that follows suit with Lyme.

I am pretty sure I speak for everyone we are CLEAR we are not doing this mess anymore!

KEY: 3 CLARITY-

Clearness of thought or style 2: a presumed capacity to perceive the truth directly and instantaneously getting clear what you really want.

If you aren't 100% completely clear what you want how will we be able to be blessed with complete healing?

I have come to the conclusion; that humans are just a confused species all together. We; as a society have gotten so accustomed to just making a buck, that we leave our own needs and God's wishes on the back burner. It is a commandment is it not that we rest on the Sabbath? God wishes us to have rest. I don't know of too many companies honoring that rule, just one thus far. (If you are a company that honors that I mean no disservice). You, think Chick-fil-A is lacking for anything? That chain is making just as much money if not more than McDonalds or other companies out there…and you know what? They are closed on Sundays to honor the Lord.   (HELLO?) Where are our priorities? Now, you need to understand my views are very diverse…this subject however, has been one source of constant frustration for me. Living life; is a beautiful, splendid gift God gave us, but it is also tiring the way we go about it. We need that day of rest, we need it to remember Our God/Source, or Universe. Remember how much we are loved, and just to re-group…to get CLARITY on our next step in life.

We have no clue what we really want, what we would LOVE to do, and walk around in a proverbial maze chasing our cheese...we can smell the cheese, yet we continually hit that wall before finally finding the opening to move forward. I can't even imagine what we must look like to God/Source etc. We are so intent on just living day to day working ourselves to the bone, to buy this and that…have to keep up with them Jones'…that we lose all site of what is really of value. We are expending so much time and energy chasing that cheese with the delusion, it is what we want and we will be able to buy this and that, when the reality really is; we are just barely surviving. The "poor" barely survive and eat, and the "wealthy" many times are empty inside still starving. (I know, I have had them as clients).

Let's put finances to the side for a few moments and talk about love; shall we? It is the same with love as well. Those who do have love; are typically not happy with the love they have, expecting the other person to make them happy, and those who don't have love are like the mice in mazes, chasing that cheese…and in the end? They aren't happy anyway. There is a reason. Lack of clarity, and lack of connection with that one Omnipresent Being…Spirit…God. My point here is we are always and forever changing our minds. Changing the mind is okay, as long as; we aren't in a constant state of doing this. Think of the mouse in the maze for a moment, he has a direction he thinks he wants to go in and he knows what he wants…that great smelling, hunk of cheese. He however hits a dead end…hits it again…and again…he works so hard and hits all the blocks. He will then try to go the other way. He changes his mind…many times, there is no follow through. It is the same with us. If you aren't 100% completely clear what you want how is God, or the Universe (should I capitalize Universe? Ah, fuck it LOL) going to be able to bless you? If you are so busy chasing that cheese, how will you hear the whisper? One more point, before we go on. We may have clarity in a situation, but we have maybe worked very hard; possibly not honoring that Sunday or for some Saturday off. Our vision, might now be happening. We begin to DOUBT and think about giving up. While; this may be a natural response, it is also not a place you want to go. The minute, you begin to doubt, this is the message God/the universe gets. Okay, so and so is giving up, they must not really want it. Now, we have to start all over. Do you see now how important this all is?

Now we will work on the clarity part.

One of the easiest and best methods for gaining clarity is cataloging or doing vision boards as known in The Secret. Cataloging as I prefer to call it, is an easy and enjoyable process that will undoubtedly help you in gaining clarity of what you desire. You can either use magazines, or printed material from computer, or any other mode you choose. I have done my best cataloging on my computer. I simply copy and paste my material into Paint or Paint Shop Pro, then save it as a .JPG and set it as the wallpaper for my computer. This method, is extremely beneficial because every time I turn on my computer or minimize screens it gets inputted into my brain, and it doesn't take up space.

You can also make better use of your cataloging by sending out positive emails for yourself.

How can this help, you may ask?

Computers have chips inside. The chips are made using quartz crystal. If it has quartz, it is an energy powerhouse and; sends out energy. I have even sent emails to myself with something I am declaring to change. I have found this method most life changing and efficient. When I send out the email to myself i.e. I am in perfect health… It then appears not only to my conscious mind, but subconscious mind as well, that it is a done deal. Sometimes; it may take a few times doing this, but it can and really has helped. If you are noticing at this stage a negative thought or impulse immediately shoot out an email to yourself stating the quote earlier.

I now take back my power and reclaim my authentic self! I am whole I am beautiful…I am at peace, and one with God/the Universe.

Do not beat yourself up, that your mind, that you, yourself; went there to that old negative and familiar place. Move forward.

Dealing with The Embarrassing Mother Fucking Relapse

That entry was written nine months ago and it was as far as I got. I stopped writing

this book for nine months…

Originally, I thought I was having a relapse and was sick again with Lyme after being

cured so "miraculously" from Stevia. Was just brain inflammation, we finally found out.

I wonder even as I type this now…"Will I ever be "normal" again?" The truth is; I am

damaged like all of you. It is very hard to relive all of this. I am doing it for you.

So, you don't feel alone…

That, after my sharing; the deepest, most secretive, part of myself, my raw,

bewildering-thoughts, the darkness I still feel…my lost…my challenges, the ones I face now in re-inventing myself…and sharing about the courage it took for me to go there…it will encourage you to still fight. That; you will FIGHT! Like a mighty warrior, knowing…someone out there, cares…that I understand your battle…and that, I believe in you, that you; can beat this!

BTW…That word originally? Was the first time I have spelled it right, since I got sick. It was the first word to go wrong for me that I couldn't spell right…VICTORY!

I have been thinking, long and hard about why I got sick. I have been asking myself this question since I knew something very bad was wrong with me. I knew if I were to completely heal myself, I had to find the root cause.

What does the Lyme bacteria do to us? It essentially eats us. So I asked myself…"What is eating me?" I started delving into the parts of my life I didn't want to remember. All those parts I just stuffed down for years since I was a child as a way; to survive it all.

I just couldn't allow this thing to rule my life like this…I couldn't allow it to take my life away. I had to do something because, it was very serious. Even though, at this point I was considered to be "Lyme free"…I wasn't. I was still suffering. I was left with PTSD, brain inflammation that was serious, and cycling back around that I "probably had MS"…"Lyme induced MS". That is just not okay for me. I can't accept that and I won't. I believe we were created to be powerful beings…and there it began.

Myself, writhing on the floor in prayer crying, and bawling like a baby.

I was entirely broken in that moment. I didn't want to live like this anymore…in this body. I didn't want to live with this brain damage, feeling ignorant, A brain that has issues spelling now, doing simple math, still stuttering when nervous or upset, tremoring, or a body that still can't bellydance! I missed my fitness that I worked so hard for…and I hated my body. I wanted my power back.

I had been on steroids, for three weeks. They pulled me off cold turkey with nothing to follow it up with. Trying to get the doctors to do anything for me was like a monkey fucking a football. All the good ones left; like a revolving door. So, there I was…alone again in this. Headaches, stabbing, eye pain…you name it I had it going wrong with me.

Including, losing my license…My boyfriend still doesn't know this.

He will when he reads this. It's humiliating…period.

I was angry. Very, very, angry. Angry at "God" "the Universe" whatever you want to call it and my faith was certainly shaken. I felt like a turtle on its back…flipped over. I was a turtle on its back flipped over. Literally. LOL There I was just lying on the floor, on my back, out of breath…waiting for the boogieman to come get me, and take me away. Then, just like that it hit me. "Go back to basics". "An aspirin a day keeps the doctor away."

I peeled myself up and off the floor, which was not an easy task. I started researching aspirin for brain inflammation. Then I remembered it also thinned blood! I had very think blood from Lyme like most of us "Lymies". If the blood is too thick it can cause huge issues for the brain. One of those being, inflammation. So, I started taking it. Slowly, I build up for a couple of days and I started feeling better. I wasn't as tired, moody, or otherwise. The tremors and ticks started going away more and my stuttering improved even when upset. My blood pressure had gone down as well, from the aspirin thinning my blood. At this point I was taking eight aspirin a day with food. There still was though, something just not right. Then I contracted two forms of pseudomonas. Back to the drawing board. I was supposed to be on Minocycline for it. I knew what I was in for if I took it and knew my brain just couldn't take it anymore. So, I went back to the Stevia. If it got rid of the Lyme maybe it would work for this. I took it until I finished the bottle again. All was well. Sort of.

The aspirin just wasn't totally cutting it for me. Not totally. There had to be something better to help my pain, my blood, and my brain. So back I went, searching the net for miracle cures for the chronic inflammation and horrid pain I was left with.

Asking questions serves a purpose, even if you ask those questions to the self.

Somehow the self knows what you need.

KEY: 4 ASK-"Lights"

For the next few Keys, the focus will be lights, camera, action. Key 4 is where the "lights" will turn on.

 Ask-

6. To expect or demand:

7. To invite:

The above definitions to ASK are the focus. I know you may be saying already, demand? Well yes, demand. Demand can be a good thing. To show this, refer to the definitions:

1. To claim as just or due:

5. Law

b. To claim formally; lay legal claim to.

All you are doing is making the rightful claim to your abundance which includes your health. It is God's, the Universes, divine desire, that you are abundant.

We are meant to be abundant in everything. It is encoded in our DNA…

There is a reason this is appearing to you in your life. Perhaps there is something you are feeling miserable about. What is eating away at you?

Are you ready now? Go ahead…

ASK!

Ask yourself, what your body needs. What do you need to get rid of? What do you need to acquire for your perfect, right, health? Take a little time with this.

So, there I was searching the net. What was it I needed? This thought kept probing my brain while searching. Then there it was.

Boswellia!

That beautiful name, from a beautiful tree, that Frankincense was made out of. For me; this has been a miracle. Not everyone can take Boswellia. Ask your body if you should take it. Remember the muscle testing? Link your fingers and pull.

I am a firm believer simple is better. If you aren't healing, ask yourself why? Go through all your meds, foods, even people you should maybe be distancing yourself from. Make a list, then get ready to…

CREATE!!!

When someone has Lyme or any other illness for that matter, it's very hard to see or acknowledge any kind of healing; because all you are dealing with is the constancy of the illness. What do we have our eye on? Do we have it on sickness or health?

That very simple question can lead to some very complex problems. Negative and positive simply cannot occupy the same space. If we are constantly focused on our illness we won't get better. There must be some positivity at the home plate for us to slide on home to.

I am sure many of you have heard the phrase, "Fake it until you make it." While it might sound like a bad sex session; it is the truth. Truth doesn't reside in fear. FEAR is just "False evidence appearing real." It isn't truth. Anything not in light or our highest good isn't our truth. If it isn't our truth no matter how shitty we might feel about getting rid of it…we need to get rid of it.

Keep in mind, I am like ya'all. I have been there…I have had the needles, IV's, been in bed for months at a time barely able to walk. Am I, perfect now? No. I had to keep tearing myself away from my misery no matter how hard it was to get back to my roots…everything I know to be true.

It is imperative, if you are to get better…you do the same thing. Even if it is just seventy seconds. It doesn't sound like much, but seventy seconds is very hard to hold positive thought to; at first. Try it. Get yourself a timer and get to work thinking positive. If you have even one miniscule negative thought, you have to start over. seventy seconds. You will hate me at first LOL; but you will love me later for it. Once you can do this…go on to the next section to create!

KEY: 5 CREATE & BELIEVE-"Camera"

Create- 4 a: to produce through imaginative skill.

Believe- b: to accept as true, genuine, or real. 2: to have a firm conviction as

to the goodness, efficacy, or ability of something--experiencing feeling.

So now that you know what you desire it is time to bring it all home. The

Universe or God gave us magnificent materials all incorporated into our bodies to help us

through life. We however, through our conditioning sometimes are not able to utilize our

brains and subconscious to their fullest capacity. Think of the brain as our physical

thinking port and our subconscious as or spiritual thinking port. They are one of the same

really with one small difference…Our subconscious is our God/Universal brain if you

will, or the brain of our soul. It is where our absolute truth lies…On an average the

average human uses only 10% of their brain and that is on a good day. It's time now to

stop wasting ourselves and start utilizing the power given us.

Remember it takes seventy seconds of pure positive thought to reprogram the brain and your subconscious. Not a lot of time however, if while focusing and visualizing, the negative creeps in you will have to start over. If you are struggling with this do not fret. I have found it is better to have even twenty seconds of pure positive thought, and visualizing without the negative creeping in, and although it takes the seventy seconds to reprogram the brain and your subconscious; here is an easy, little thing to help. In most pet shops they have training clickers. Just stick with me here on this…

Just as your camera captures that picture; that is reflected into its lens, into its memory banks, as does your brain and subconscious with the outside world. So, if you have had issues making it to the seventy seconds mark, get a clicker and click it after twenty seconds or so. Your brain and subconscious will be programmed up to that point and you can continue further each time, until you have gotten to the seventy seconds. This method will save you a lot of frustration. Once you are there at the finish line again, click your clicker. You will be amazed with the results.

We are going to now visualize and create the feeling within ourselves so that we are in total alignment with God/the Universe. Be sure you are calm and have done the previous exercises mentioned first.

You can use a timer if you need to and sometimes it helps with keeping the mind clear of the negativity. Pay close attention to the visuals and what you are telling yourself. Repeat until you have completed seventy seconds of pure positive thought and visualizing on any one certain project.

Please note that, the seventy second exercise was taught to me. I however, at first had such an issue getting in there it took up a good two minutes to get rid of the stink. It takes sixty-eight seconds to transform any negative into positive. So, use the seventy second mark. When you can complete this move onto the next section. Keep some notes on the next page of your progress.

Notes

How'd you do?

Chapter 7 The Climax

I think that no matter what our religion; everyone enjoys a good climax! (I know I do.)

LOL. Agreed? You are there now. Get ready for the delivery. Well, this has nothing to do

with sex. Your mind however, went there…you dirty bird. LOL. See, that took all of

about seventy seconds.

Let's look at what the definition of climax is:

2a :the highest point: culmination

-       the *climax* of a distinguished career
b :the point of highest dramatic tension or a major turning point in the action (as
of a play)

3:a relatively stable ecological stage or community especially of plants that is
achieved through successful adaptation to an environment; *especially* :the final
stage in ecological succession

Going back to my boyfriend for a few minutes. He taught me everything about a good

climax. Again, nothing to do with sex. He is the highest, most admirable man, I have ever

met in my life. He, makes me feel things…that I can't even begin to comprehend or

explain. He is the highest of all highs, if ever there was one. I adore him, so fervently,
with so much…fire and passion; it just can't ever be explained by all the words in the
English language, though I try to; with an obsession LOL.

Before, you all go; "this chick is off her rocker…"LOL Yes, you are right in many
ways; I am. We all are, a little; after Lyme, aren't we?

Here's the thing, and where this is SO; relevant.

I had a 186 IQ; before I got Lyme as stated before. I think…I forgot if I did or not.
HA! I never did anything with it LOL. I had babies. Which was great, and wonderful, and
everything wild, that follows. However, this man; and what he caused within myself
during one of the darkest, moments of my life, is the reason I am even alive, and writing
this book, possibly making you laugh. He is the embodiment of all climaxes; and
everything good and holy.

Due; to his undying patience with me; when I acted crazy, neurotic, and everything in-
between…he stayed by my side, even though he might not have understood, directly; just

what I was going through. He could have left. However, because he chose to stay and

support me; I found an even better, part of myself; I didn't realize I even had.

He is, why; again, I am writing this book for you…even if it's just for laughter.

You say; okay, okay… enough about him how will this help me?

This will help you, because; you are going to fall in love.

WITH YOURSELF!

It, will help you; because so many of us, lose ourselves during this vicious, bitch of a

MOFO, disease. I did all this stuff I am writing about; over and over, and with his

undying love.

I will be your girlfriend, your boyfriend; and help you to fall in love…

With yourself.

When you have been able to grasp everything, I have said; move on to the next step.

Peace.

KEY: 6 DELIVERY-"Action"

Delivery-1. a freeing from an obligation or responsibility.

The above definition should give you a great sense of satisfaction. This is where now you no longer; have, to worry…you no longer take this on. You know all is well and all is taken care of. You KNOW you have already received your abundance, your health.

Now…This is also where it may be confusing. Remember back on KEY 4 when I mentioned God's/ the Universe's timing? It may not appear to you quite yet but it doesn't mean it is not there, or it may have appeared to you as signs. Yet, there is this KNOWING that is undeniable, and you aren't sure why you know it you just do.

This "Key" my friends, is all about letting go; about your climax. You are freeing yourselves, from the responsibility and allowing it to happen; because you KNOW without a doubt, that it will happen. You no longer have to worry about tomorrow or what it will bring because you know it will all be good. It is when now you will be waking in the morning with a pure and open heart instead of the same old "Oh great now I have to get up."

You may now ask me as everyone before "Well…How do I let go? What is it like, and how do I know it has happened?" Perhaps, you have tried to let go before and yet no matter what you tried to do nothing seemed to work. It is not your fault you just didn't have the tools or anything to compare it to. Are you ready for the answer? Turn the page…

Remember back when we were working on your energy field and your chakras? When you were doing the breathing exercise and you felt that coldish kind of breeze? It is very similar to that experience. This is the "lock and load" moment…It is however, a lot more intense than that mild breeze. You will get chills all over…it is undeniable….it is very similar in sensation to having an orgasm. That's right, I said it. That is what it is like… When you are visualizing everything happening, and being in that state of gratitude you start becoming so elated, so excited at your new life; you start getting "chills", all those butterflies, perhaps even tears of joy that finally, finally, finally, you have completed your first mission!

If some of you are still having issues with this then I have a solution. Visualize, and create while you are approaching orgasm. I realize to some it may sound blasphemous. It is not meant to be offensive or ridiculous, but it is a natural function of our bodies, and

we should be comfortable with it. It is a beautiful thing when you are in that moment of

being with God/ the Universe and in that place of gratitude. It is not a bad thing…and for

some this is what works, at least at first, until you get the hang of letting go. This is a

place that a lot of people are seriously lacking in their lives and it was not meant to lie

dormant; for several, seasons at a time. This is not meaning to go get several partners,

and have as many orgasms "to create". You don't need a partner for this and it is best in

fact if you don't. Learn to love being alone with your body. It is sacred; and that is the

whole point.

For right now work with this Key for a week or so before you move on to Key 7.

KEY: 7 RECEIVE-"Celebration"

Receive- 2 a: to act as a receptacle or container for--b: to assimilate-(1 a: to take in and utilize as nourishment: absorb into the system b: to take into the mind and thoroughly comprehend through the mind or senses).

Well, you have made it. Good job! Give yourself a firm pat on the back. It's time to count all ten fingers and all ten toes of your beautiful creation. In Key 7 we will talk about celebrating life. By now you should have a good idea at least, that being joyful and happy gets you much further in life than being in a constant state of being angry, depressed, or in misery. Have you ever gone out somewhere just to watch people? I have, and have gone as much as eight hours; without seeing one single person smile! This is a sad state, of affairs indeed.

We were meant to be happy and joyful.

Here I will quote the Bible:

In Ecclesiastes 3:1 it states…To everything there is a season, and a time to every purpose under the heaven.

In verse 4 A time to weep, and a time to laugh; a time to mourn, and a time to dance…

I am not telling you that you should never feel sadness or anger…to feel these emotions is human. I am merely saying feel it and let it go and be joyful for a new day. Each and every day I am reminded how great God/and the Universe is; for my family, and my beautiful, lovely, darling, man…and how much I am loved.

This doesn't mean I don't have challenges still. I have so many; like so many of you. I might always be this way. Hard to tell yet.

However, I look back at my life. Back at a time when I was like many of you…angry, filled with hate for myself, for others, with absolutely no joy. I was so busy feeling that anger, I wasn't enjoying life. It makes me so grateful where I am now and for the support I have from God/the Universe, and yes…for my boyfriend; my other universe…LOL.

This has not come to me however, without work on my part. I had to allow the joy to come to me and fill me up. That's the great part of this last step, all it takes is the willingness to rest, to sit and take it in…and be the receptacle.

The author of Ecclesiastes goes on to speak about what may be one of the most profound and important lessons besides the resurrection; miracle of Jesus.

They state in Ecclesiastes 3:9-13:

9What profit hath he that worketh in that wherein he laboureth?

10I have seen the travail, which God hath given to the sons of men to be exercised in it.

11He hath made everything beautiful in his time: also he hath set the world in their heart, so that no man can find out the work that God maketh from the beginning to the end.

12I know that there is no good in them, but for a man to rejoice, and to do good in his life.

13And also that every man should eat and drink, and enjoy the good of all his labour, it is the gift of God.

Now, how many of us enjoy the fruits of our labors? So many of us "Lymies" have certainly labored. How many of us have done things for ourselves lately?

Many of us have worked from sun up to sun down and past…For many of us our home is our work. We say we work so we can live, but is that really living? Working so hard, sometimes barely eating (how ironic), just to make that buck…so we can hmmmm eat? So, we can enjoy "the finer things in life". Yet, we aren't enjoying life because we are too busy working too hard trying to keep up with the Jones's or idea of what living

really is; or too busy being sick.

Take time out…Smell the flowers, walk barefoot on the grass, mothers and fathers

enjoy the fruits of our labors our children…They are only young for a season…Life is

only here for a season. So, take it in, take all of it in, all of it…even the adversity and

embrace it…breathe it all in…embrace each and every day God has given you…receive,

celebrate, and rejoice in it.

I am just going to mention a few other points I feel are important, with biblical reference listed first.

1.

{1 Timothy 4:16

16Take heed unto thyself, and unto the doctrine; continue in them: for in doing this thou shalt both save thyself, and them that hear thee.}

I would like you to keep in mind that our lives are likened to that of a movie. If you don't keep your mind on it, if you don't just get quiet within yourself, you are likely to miss important plot points. This then puts you at risk with the deer in the headlights complex, causing you to possibly feel lost; with no direction whatsoever, and even forlorn with your life.

I can't begin to stress the importance for you to on a daily basis, to make a commitment to yourself and do the upkeep to keep yourself in check. Surround yourself with people that mirror the new you, and make the time for spiritual pursuits, for you, and the things that hold importance. If you have a hard time doing this yourself, find a spiritual mentor for a time, allowing yourself the funds (if they are needed) and the time to meet with them, because you are worth it.

2.

{Proverbs 23:7

7For as he thinketh in his heart, so is he: Eat and drink, saith he to thee; but his heart is not with thee.}

{Proverbs 14:30

30A sound heart is the life of the flesh: but envy the rottenness of the bones.}

We are going to discuss the difference between our conscious mind and subconscious mind.

Our conscious mind changes thoughts and acts like a conductor or director if you will, and sends the information to the subconscious "actors" and the subconscious then "acts" out the direction then reflecting it back out into our outside world. Something doesn't have to be going on in our outside world for this to happen and become "reality". It can happen with just one single little thought.

Our conscious mind utilizes only approximately 10% of its capacity and our subconscious uses 90%. Quite a difference… When you utilize both together and are always in this "awareness" state; both become merged and act as a very powerful conductor… Think 200%.

Conscious Mind=Physical "Body" Mind || Subconscious Mind=God/Universal "Soul" Mind.

"You have a very powerful mind that can make anything happen as long as you keep yourself centered." Dr. Wayne W. Dyer

This subconscious mind; your "soul's brain", is what really runs everything, or tries to.

"We either make ourselves miserable, or we make ourselves strong. The amount of work is the same." Carlos Castaneda

Here is another analogy…

When we take a picture with a camera, light reflected from the object we see with our eyes passes through the shutter, diaphragm, and lens ("eyes") and form a real, inverted image. The "nano" second during which the shutter is open, this image imbeds onto the surface of the film "our subconscious" causing an invisible image to be recorded into it.

Our "film" section in the brain is almost, at the beginning of the optic radiation part of the brain towards the "Wernicke's Area." This "film" section is directly related to our "subconscious". When we visualize, the brain doesn't know the difference between visually seeing it, with our eyes or otherwise. Our subconscious "sees" and acknowledges it as reality.

Picture on next page of the brain.

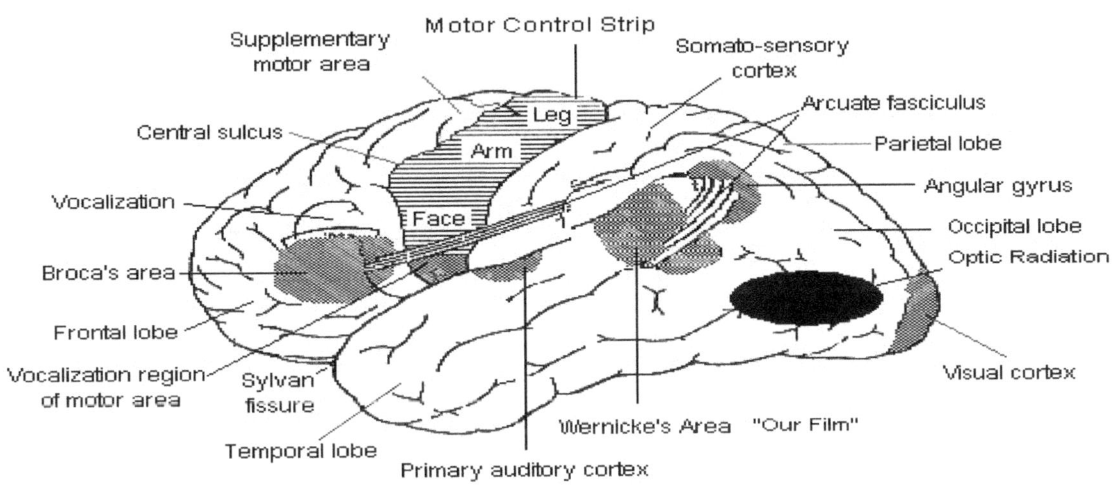

This is why; it is so important for us to watch what we say and how we view things. All of it, every bit of it is recorded.

If I had ten cents for every time I said OMG I am so sick; I'd be a millionaire.

If we have a negative thought "click" goes the camera and it is perceived as real.

The same goes for a positive thought..."click" and "reality."

3.

{Psalm 33:3

3Sing unto him a new song; play skillfully with a loud noise.}

It is so important to feel some "drive" for something. When we are driven to complete any task, it makes the path so much more enjoyable, and much easier. All drive means, is getting excited, forging through no matter what and not letting anything stop you. When we feel drive towards something, it can give us a sense of purpose and a feeling like our time here means something…Ya' know? Much like my boyfriend. LOL

SO

GET

EXCITED!

and…he does excite me so much!

As I mentioned earlier in the book, take time out to notice all the beauty around you. Get excited about waking up in the morning, and if you must pretend for a bit until you get it, so be it.

Just as if you were a child again and filled with; carefree play…Pretend!

4.

{1 Corinthians 14:40 (King James Version)

40 Let all things be done decently and in order.}

Now it's time to get organized. Easier said than done. Especially with Lyme.

So many of us have issues with this one…I know I have. I have noticed this more with people who have a lot of creative ability; and those who are very analytical. Our minds go so much, that we tend to get ahead of ourselves, starting way too many projects at once then we get overloaded trying to keep up. Sound familiar?

I have found what helps the most, is when I have a budding idea I make a note of it, maybe take time out with a few sentences on it, put it in a file of its own, and put it away.

I will then go back to the original project and work on it until completed. Sometimes, I might take a break from the original project at hand, look it over and maybe see how I can perfect it, or go through my other projects and if I get any ideas and make notes, or a sketch should it come to mind. These are only ideas and not actually embarking full on.

"When you have that "#boreowhateveritfuckingis' rummaging through your body; you can't concentrate on anything!!! Let's face it we are lucky, if we even remember to go to the bathroom.

I feel it is important to take a few minutes when these ideas come up and jot them down. Just make sure you go back to the original project until it is completed. Then pat yourself on the back for a job well done, and move on to the next. It makes all the difference in the world.

"Even if it is just a few minutes spent on one project."

5.

{Hebrews 11:1 (King James Version)

1Now faith is the SUBSTANCE of things hoped for, the

EVIDENCE of things not seen.}

In the Bible the word substance is not highlighted. I highlighted it to point out the "meat" in this verse, and it is how I have always personally felt about faith for myself. I cannot begin to tell you, how many times I have been persecuted for having "faith" in things not seen by others. I had this faith because God/the Universe has either shown me or told me himself; about certain things to come in my life. God/the Universe has told me it is my right to be fruitful in all things; so why on earth would I not trust that?

You will also notice I have highlighted evidence. These two words are physical. We know in the English language that these two words mean something tangible and physical. Something you can hang on to, something that nourishes you.

{Evidence: Idiom: in evidence

1.   Plainly visible; to be seen}

{Substance:

1. a. That which has mass and occupies space; matter.

2. b. Gist; heart.} *

Call me crazy but if something has mass and occupies space it is physical. This means it is "real". If evidence means, even in idiom; "plainly visible" than this also brings a sense of "reality" to faith.

Whew…what a relief; I am not crazy after all!

Faith moves mountains…

{Matthew 19:26 (King James Version)

26 But Jesus beheld them, and said unto them, with men this is impossible;

but with God all things are possible.}

I am going to share with you a story. This story can be medically validated.

I was once told by a "doctor", I would never have children. HA!!! SNORTING!!! If I did get pregnant, I would surely miscarriage, as I had too much scaring on my uterus. (rape related).

Four children later, I was sure; I was pregnant. I was sicker than a dog. I however was not late and having heavy periods. Pregnancy tests were not accurate.   One positive one negative. I went to the doctor; they did a serum blood test and negative. So, they did an ultrasound and saw no baby.

About a month had passed and I was still very sick and throwing up. I went back to the doctor (still having periods) they did another blood test HCG was elevated but not enough to say positive and they thought that maybe I had cancer. I began praying. I had faith…I bought little girl baby socks and shirt and carried it with me everywhere. I was still sick and a month later went back to the doctor. Another blood test, the HCG was raised a little but not enough for a "viable pregnancy". They thought I still had cancer and did another ultra sound. They saw a "mass" in my uterus and said if it were a fetus there would be a heart beating there. And that the "mass" had to be removed.

I refused. I knew with all that I was I was pregnant. How? God/the Universal being told me. Why would I not believe? They all thought I was minus a few straws. Some more time passed, and the local doctor sent me to a specialist. This had been a stressful situation for me so a friend went with me for moral support to the specialist. The technician says to me "I am really sorry Maam', I see the baby there's the heart but it is not moving. The baby is not alive." Tears filled my eyes. The young male tech not knowing what to do left the room. I started getting up to get dressed to leave, when the tech walks back in and says, "Why don't we try something…" he had two cranberry juices and two apple juices and two Snickers bars. He instructed me to eat them as fast as I could and then drink 32 oz. of water and walk briskly around the hospital and come back in fifteen minutes. I did as instructed.

He puts the goop on my belly and tried and tried talking to the baby that was clearly having no heartbeat. I crying, and hysterical started praying like I had never prayed before. The technician says again "Maam, I am very sorry…" He almost looked more forlorn than me. He was just going to take off the paddle when my friend exclaims "LOOK!" That little baby was swirling so fast and furious in a circle… round and round she went, then stopped. Behold... a heartbeat. The poor tech…wide eyed hand on head, congratulated me and away I went with my paper in hand that I was pregnant. I had an appointment with my doctor that week and when he looked at the ultrasound, he said again there was no heartbeat. I saw it too no heartbeat. He still wanted to do a DNC because he was sure something was wrong with the baby. No heart beat nothing.

I couldn't do it…God told me I was pregnant and therefore I was. They thought I was nuts. Two month later the doc did an ultrasound and well would you look at that, the heart was beating! I was six and a half months pregnant at that point and she came a month later. She was tiny but she was beautiful, sassy, and fine. Not a thing wrong with her.

Except, her sassy attitude now. LOL

I shared this with you, because it proves faith has SUBSTANCE to it.

Faith itself is a living thing, and has a life all of its own. This means, we can help our bodies heal from this voracious, asshole, of a disease.

Never doubt that things can turn around for you, no matter what the issue may be.

I am quoting again…

{Matthew 19:26 (King James Version)

26 But Jesus beheld them, and said unto them, with men this is impossible;

but with God all things are possible.}

SIMPLE…FIN.

6.

{James 5:13

...Meeting Specific Needs...

13Is any among you afflicted? let him pray. Is any merry? let him sing psalms.}

In these days of the world, I cannot stress enough the importance of setting aside separate, time with God. So many of us ignore this importance and don't call upon God or spend any time with him until we are in an emergency situation, and need immediate gratification. Only then do we call out with stupendous fervor "My Lord My God" …We seem content for whatever reason living a mediocre life, just going through the motions of everyday life. In the Bible it says God is a jealous God…I don't necessarily believe this…I do believe however, God/the Universe is a protective God/Father/universal love; and cares about his creations.

Just as we as parents and creators care about our children, our creations…we want to spend time with the people and things we love, yes? As does God or whatever your "unit of love is". Just time made saying "Hey YOU, it has been a fucked-up day for me; just checking in." This gives so much pleasure to the one light; the one who created us. God/the Universe; always, always returns the favor…ALWAYS. I think many feel God/whoever it is for you, doesn't need us, that God doesn't need anything. Not only does God need us, God hungers for you, pines for us. God lives and breathes for us. God/that universal love; desires our presence; every minute of every day.

I look around at our society…God is being removed from everything…people seem to be afraid of God, so afraid they are removing God from the school systems and monuments. God, is quickly becoming a name that isn't socially acceptable.

Why?

Children; love God. I was not brought up in a Christian household, yet I knew exactly who God was and I knew he made me happy. Not only do we need to be seeking God out; spending special time with Him/Her/It, we need to be teaching our children to do the same.

I'll be honest with you…I have cussed out "God" many times after Lyme.

Dude…sometimes it was bad! LOL

I am still standing…I wasn't struck down by lightening; and I still healed from Lyme.

Just saying.

It is the whole point; of being here on this earth…realizing we are not separate from God/that universal love. The only way to learn this though, is through spending time with Him/Her/It.

I am going to mention one more point here. I am sure you have noticed I refer to God as Him. God is to you, who you need Him to be. I grew up without a father. This is what I needed…it is what was provided for me. Perhaps you are someone who grew up without a mother, God is versatile. God can mother as well. If you have any question about the existence of God, as I mentioned earlier in this book…Ask God to shower you with His love…It, I promise you is undeniable; and fucking overwhelming, beautiful! Yes, much like my boyfriend. LOL

I am closing with a quote from Brennan Manning (Not many people know of him):

"I am now utterly convinced, that on judgment day the Lord Jesus is going to ask us one question and only one question…Did you believe that I loved you? That I desired you? That I waited for you day after day? That I longed to hear the sound of your voice?"

I say to you…Do You? Never, ever doubt how important you are to God.

It is very hard; I realize, when you have something like Lyme…to believe; God/universal love, loves you. I have been there so many times. However…

This book has brought be back to this; at least in the now…Thank you.

{Colossians 3:23

23And whatsoever ye do, do it **HEARTILY**, as to the Lord, and not unto men.}

HEARTILY = Enthusiastic- Adjective 1. Having or showing great excitement and interest.

Yeah; well, when one has Lyme…that shit goes right down the fucking toilet!

How many of us live our lives this way? Even those not sick? As I mentioned earlier, we are meant to love what we do for work. God/Christ/that universal love, does not wish for us to be miserable at what we do. It is even a commandment to keep the Sabbath holy. How many of us remember to do that? How many of us; look for that in work as a prerequisite of the work place, in order to be blessed by THAT presence? Many corporations refuse to honor this.

I know that this may be a scary thought for some, but if you are not happy in your work you need to change that. It may be a matter of you growing closer to God, or you may need to change your work place. Regardless where your issue might be; it is something you need to pay attention to and honor in your own life. Working yourself to the bone, for the sake of the almighty dollar, so you can "live" is not living. It is dying.

{Proverbs 23:4

4Labour not to be rich: cease from thine own wisdom.}

"This means also with Lyme…dare to be unconventional."

8.

There are a few verses from the bible to be the focus of this section. This is maybe the most important. I know where all of you might be. I have been there. I have been so damned angry I got sick and everything I have lost because of Lyme. At times it just doesn't seem fair. The decaying process our bodies go through, the attitudes of others while we are going through this; between the doctors, sometimes our family and friends…just, makes this illness unbearable at times. It's easy to start hating our bodies, and ourselves.

However, if we are hateful to ourselves how will our body heal like it needs to?

{Matthew 22:37-39

37Jesus said unto him, thou shalt love the Lord thy God with all thy heart, and with all thy soul, and with all thy mind.

38This is the first and great commandment.

39And the second is like unto it, thou shalt love thy neighbor as thyself.}

How many of us though, love ourselves? Especially with Lyme. What are your feelings about your body, right now this minute as you read this? Take a few minutes to write that in the space here:

{Luke 10:25-28

The Parable of the Good Samaritan:

25And, behold, a certain lawyer stood up, and tempted him, saying, Master, what shall I

do to inherit eternal life?

26He said unto him, what is written in the law? how readest thou?

27And he answering, said, Thou shalt love the Lord thy God with all thy heart, and with all thy soul, and with all thy strength, and with all thy mind; and thy neighbor as thyself.

28And he said unto him, thou, hast answered right: this do, and thou shalt live."}

{Proverbs 25:21

21If thine enemy be hungry, give him bread to eat; and if he be thirsty, give him water to drink:}

{Matthew 5:44

44But I say unto you, love your enemies, bless them that curse you, do good to them that hate you, and pray for them which despitefully use you, and persecute you.}

This one section, may be the single most important…We don't realize that when we curse our enemies, when we wish bad for our enemies, it only harms us not them. This includes our illness. To not be at peace is a sad thing indeed. To not be at peace with yourself…that is a tragedy. I have been on the opposite side before…I am not perfect, and because I have been there on that alternative side, and experienced life on both sides of the spectrum, I know what works and what doesn't. Feeling spite and animosity for anything does absolutely, no good to your life and can even bring on sickness.

Ask yourself what was going on in my life when I got sick? Make a note of it. For some of you it's a job you hate, perhaps you aren't taking enough time for yourself, your family. Maybe, the ending of a relationship, an ex, perhaps we have a challenging family...perhaps you are mad at yourself for not writing, or following some dream.

I am absolutely convinced the only way out of any illness is to love everything. All in love with everything. People, places, things…your illness. Yup, even the mother fucking illness. LOL. The only way to anything good and worthwhile is through love. If you want to create good in your life, if you want to heal your body, it is as simple as this, LOVE everything…and, LOVE yourself.

Right here make some notes some different ways, you can start being kind to yourself:

9.

{Mark 11:24-

24Therefore I say unto you, What things so ever ye desire, when ye pray, believe that ye

receive them, and ye shall have them.}

I wonder so many times how many of us, believe. Believe in anything, God/Universe,

miracles, or that you are loved. We were all made, our souls from a beautiful image. A

big, beautiful, bold, powerful force. This same magnetizing, powerful force in within us.

We have, this intrinsic power within us just waiting to be unleashed. All this power; and

yet no one even begins to tap into it. We are instead convinced so many of us, that we are

powerless…especially with Lyme. I have been there myself, remember?

In a synopsis for a poetry book I wrote before this, I stated that: "It is truly amazing

these poems arrived out of myself. Through a very jumbled and damaged brain, sick in

bed for months at a time, barely able to walk and talk, and sometimes barely able to see.

Even now, as I type this…it brings tears to my eyes. It was hell on earth…feeling like you are confined to a fish bowl with no water, looking out. Aware of what's going on with your body, and the feeling of powerlessness that you can do nothing about it except lay in defeat." YOU…ARE…NOT…DEFEATED!

The truth is YOU are POWERFUL!

If you don't really believe in yourself, in your healing, how can your body heal?

Whether it's from the Bible, "For as he thinketh in his heart, so is he" or whether it's coming from the Law of Attraction; it's all the same.

What is your heart thinking about your body right now? Write is here:

Think about this for a minute, if you don't believe things can change for you it goes against both Universal Law and God's Law. This makes us unreachable, and we are just too damned valuable to allow something like this to happen.

Almost from the beginning of time, we have known somehow that by two it places so much more value into whatever it may be in that moment. When we believe in something, when we really believe, miracles can happen.

My boyfriend doesn't realize the magnitude, that his presence, has had on my life…because he believed in me, and taught me; to believe in myself.

Belief in something, really, believing in something; is like being in love. It is a very powerful magnetizing force. When you love yourself, when you believe in yourself, you become so powerful!

Positive and negative; simply can't live in the same space. It's like magnets rubbing against each other.

A lot of us may also think we believe but do we really? Visualize you have a one-hundred-dollar bill in your hand. Do you really believe; it is there, or do those nagging thoughts start coming that you don't really have it? "Well, there isn't really one hundred in my hand." Just because you can't see something, doesn't mean it's not there. We, all know this from Lyme…this includes our healing.

"I am in perfect, right, health!"

Say it! Say it with fervor like being in love. Make this your personal mantra and recite it repeatedly; until you believe it.

I have had gemstones fall "out of nowhere" in my car into my lap, that when taken to a crystal shop and jewelers they could not classify it. I have sat down and really believed with all that I am that I was blessed right now in that moment with five hundred dollars.

I'll walk outside and there it is in my yard.

I will quote again…

{Mark 11:24-

24Therefore I say unto you, What things so ever ye desire, when ye pray, believe that ye receive them, and ye shall have them.}

Whether your belief system is from the Bible, or metaphysical in nature…just believe. That should be a t-shirt for all of us" Just believe!"

Believe in yourself, that you can heal your body, and believe that perfect, right, health is yours now! Spend some time on this over the next few days, before you go on to the next section.

10.

{Proverbs 16:3-

3Commit thy works unto the LORD,

and thy thoughts shall be established.}

What a great promise that is! It really doesn't get any better than that. Make a commitment, (work hard and stay on task) is all that means and yet we are so rebellious against it. Why, I wonder? Perhaps, it is because it is requested that we are committing ourselves to something. Humans don't like commitment…and especially commitment to the self. Whew, that's a big responsibility, the self.

Your body is a beautiful temple! Say it! LOL

(I'm snorting laughter, scoffing when I say this myself now. LOL)

We are all in the same place.

How many of us are committed to ourselves? Are you committed to yourself?

Are you committed to your healing, or are you chasing it? Think about that for a minute. There is a huge difference. Being committed to your healing means relaxing, breathing, taking time out…and being kind to ourselves. Most of us "Lymies" are like mice in a maze; chasing that stupid, chunk, of cheese. We are so focused and fixated on the illness to the point of abandoning ourselves.

Stop chasing, and start committing to being kind and loving to yourself.

I believe in you that you can do it!

11.

{Job 3:25-

25For the thing which I greatly feared is come upon me, and that which I was afraid of is

come unto me.}

FEAR

False Evidence Appearing Real

There is no such thing as negativity. Negativity is not real it is false. It is simply the

absence of truth, and who makes your truth? You do. If something is seemingly negative,

and creeping up in your life, think *stop, drop, and roll*. The point of this is, changing the

current then take a good look, chuckle, and say well wasn't that interesting?

All things *negative, appearing* as *real;* are actually, positive. It brings about necessary change. Embrace it and give thanks…even to our "appeared" illness.

It ultimately doesn't matter what is troubling you today. If you can just absorb and *know* that whatever seems to be negative, is merely the absence of truth, you will begin to realize your right truth, and you can make that truth manifest. Including your perfect right health.

12.

We all know having Lyme, makes us just want to leave our bodies…and just escape. However, if we leave our bodies; we can't heal ourselves effectively. Grounding is very important to implement while we are here. When we aren't grounded we tend to be accident prone and it can cause even fatal accidents, and even illness. It also connects us to Source or Heavenly Father and helps us to not feel that separation. However, it is not just about being grounded.

Ephesians 3:15-19 Specifically 3:17 {17 That Christ may dwell in your hearts by faith; that ye **being rooted and grounded in love**,}

Love is a very big, again, magnetizing force. Nothing bad can live in love. The below exercise is to help you begin to be grounded in love.

Grounding Exercise

There are a few different methods for this. Some see themselves rooted into the ground like a tree, others with light. Ultimately it is all the same. Your soul has to be rooted, not just rooted, rooted in love. Here are the procedures, I have found to be the best. At first it may seem like a lot of work, but before you know it; it will be instantaneous. The first time I grounded myself it took me three hours. This doesn't mean it will take you that long but it gives you an indication how absent I used to be from my own life.

Make sure you begin with breathing. Breathing is essential in any healing, and many of us don't breathe correctly when we are ill.

Step 1. Close your eyes. Breathe in your nose and out your mouth, (breathing through your diaphragm) slowly and deliberately releasing any negativity you may have from your day.

Repeat 5x.

Step 2. Breathe in your nose and out your nose again breathing from your diaphragm. Breathe as slow as is comfortable.

Repeat 5x.

Keeping your eyes closed:

Visualize a big bright sun over the top of your head feel its warmth.

At the bottom of the sun is a silver cord.

Start pulling cord down through your head to your neck…

Through your chest…

Through your abdomen…

Through your genitals…

Splitting the cord into two still silver.

Put into each thigh and go down to the knees…

Through the knees…

Through your calves…

Through your ankles...

Through your feet… (your feet may start to feel heavy, extreme heat, or tingly)

Push this cord to the very center of the earth.

Wrap this cord around and secure by any means you visualize.

You may notice tingling in other places of your body, and things may seem brighter to you and possibly even clearer as if you were wearing glasses.

Should this method not work for you, some of the kids I have worked with have seen themselves as a lightning rod and brought down electricity from the sun all the way through the center of the earth.

Either way is effective, or you may even "be given" another method for you that is easier. If your feel heavy, tingly, or otherwise you know it has worked.

Onward we go acquiring your magnificence, go on to the next page.

13.

Maintaining Your Flexibility and Gaining Back Your Magnificence

This was born due to my body needing more flexibility and oxygen. At one point I was a very, very, large woman. I am not very coordinated to begin with LOL and at this point in my life I couldn't do Yoga to save my life. I am not convinced that the human body is supposed to do all those poses and even knew a yoga instructor who faced losing her business and her health until this was given to her. She has since incorporated it into her daily classes and her body has since healed. Originally, I came up with the name Ojasvitaa which is a Sanskrit name. It means magnificence.

Get very acquainted with your breath as in the exercise previously before doing this. Your joints need oxygen going through them to work properly and maintain flexibility.

With bottoms of feet touching each other palms of hands facing up resting on knees.

Breathe in through nose count of 5

And raise right arm up over head one side with back of hand facing left.

Hold breath for a count of 5 raising other arm same as other side touching backs of hands.

Turn palms of hands and place them together exhaling slowly through mouth bringing hands down slowly Namaste position with elbows level to wrist.

Now left arm. Repeat cycle 6 times total rotating right arm then left arm.

Cup feet first right hand then left. Start breathing in nose slow, deep and steady, bringing body down gently and allow body to fall where it wants naturally do not force this.

Steady breaths in nose out nose.

Breathing 5 complete breaths in nose and out before beginning next cycle.

Do this 5x

Listen to your body. Only do what is comfortable. If you cannot hold your breath for count of 5, do only what is comfortable for you even if it is a count of 1 or 2. You will get there. If your body can only handle 1 or 2 times a week honor your body's needs. Try to increase weekly. Again, if you can't increase weekly, increase every two weeks. Take your time this is not a contest.

Poems from My Battle with Lyme Disease

Sometimes; I detest who I have come to be...

Someone, who appears weak; not strong...

Someone, who is like a hermit crab; crushable with one mighty step...

   if you spent just a fraction; of a fortnight in my shoes...

I think that then; I might amaze you...

   and then you would wonder...

However; I made it through...

   and I would answer most earnestly...

It was because of beautiful; you...

I held your beauty within my visual field; until I could make it real for me...

I held your strength in my heart; until I could roar voraciously...

Even though I appear weak; I am mighty and strong...

I have not given up; and I draw my sword...

   yet, I am still; and allow them to feed on me...

For you are my flesh, my bread, my wine; my communion...

   and "they" the indomitable "Greens"; cannot get to me.

Force of Nature

Who knows how long the locusts have been eating away at me?

  turned me from a mighty, little tree, to a weak stem; a sucker...

To have so much of myself stripped away; so painful...

Yet; I am expected to carry on, even though I am nothing but a weed, a burden...

  diseased...

The grandest tree, with the greatest roots, and sunflower heart...

My greatest, sweetest dream; seems lost somewhere in the forest...

All it would have taken was the slightest of care; at a most delicate time...

  from anyone; to help me grow into a beautiful redwood...

Right when my roots were finally taking hold; when I was a new sapling...

A trunk all my own...

A treat of nature; full of pleasantness, sweet scent and musky aroma...

Just getting her first rings...

Beautiful buds...

The "Greens" disguised as a beautiful meadow; in the forest of your heart...

Latched themselves onto me...

Diseased me...

The soil all around me turned into a vast ocean; no nourishment; only when convenient
from the seasons...

Your heart; the most beautiful forest...

Floated further and further away; from the elements...

Distanced, seemingly by continents; yet were right next to me...

I kept sending out the signals from my very best buds...

Again, a sucker, to weak stem, to diseased seed...

To the larvae of the locusts; eating away at me...

Yet, inside me the pith; it lives...

It remembers when we met and I began to grow backwards...

I saw you and grew buds...

I grew branches and roots...

My outer bark became dead to what was before...

My inner bark; it lived for you...

My cambian; it grew for you...

My ray; it felt for you...

My sapwood; it lovingly fed you when I myself was dry...

In my feeding you; extractives were formed...

My heartwood; it became strong and rich!

  but my pith; even when you weren't looking...

Kept its original eye on you...

  and is still sprouting...

My heartwood is still intact...

The extractives are still formed...

I am still feeding you; in feeding you it feeds me...

I still feel for you...

I still dare to grow for you...

I still live for you...

Which protects the heartwood; rich and strong...

My branches are still there reaching for you...

My buds and blossoms; still send their signal to you...

I remember when we began to grow...

   and the seed was planted...

Suddenly; I am no longer diseased...

Again, without even knowing...

A force of nature...

You planted me; and I am again...

Alive; and...

I am strong; in you...

My beautiful force of nature.

Come on in and sit a spell where the "Greens" do not roam...

Just you; just me...

Beautiful, normalcy...

I've been fighting this so long; I've forgotten who I am...

Not much left to my beautiful, originality; just you...

You the last remnant, before the "Greens" took over...

To my beauty...

My independence...

Myself...

You; beautiful you...

Mirror me; beautiful me...

Before the "Greens" took over...

Splendicity.

The touch of you, haunts my soul; in the very deepest of ways…

In the same way, a forest has been abandoned; waiting for the gods to water…

As I lay here in my scorched earth; reaching for you my oxygen…

Love me again; recurrently…

So, my leaves will sprout again.

You fill me up; you fill up my senses...

From diseased tree; make me feel new...

You make me feel beauty reclaimed...

fresh blossoms with new morning dew...

You make me feel spring tide; life growing again...

Fractured Fairy Tale

The gem inside still shines so bright for beautiful you...

It's the only beauty left to me underneath the "Lymie" hues...

I feel like an ogre hidden in a cave underneath this "Lymie" hide...

and that no one sees or acknowledges the princess I still am inside...

I don't want to be in this body anymore; "Lymie" defining who I am...

I'd rather be remembered "the best woman ever" in all the land...

Take the sword from the stone each layer gently cut...

Take the gem before the "Greens" steal it too; leaving me a hollow trunk...

Take the gem for yourself; for beautiful you...

It's the only life left to me underneath the "Lymie" hues.

I reach out to you when the miserable hits; It's hell fighting this alone...

the abnormalities surmounting...

the realities lingering...

My merry go round; constantly moving...

no one can catch me...

I can't see my focal point...

Everyone needs one in times of grim; that one thing that extracts...

the strength to fight...

the beauty still encompassed within...

You are my beauty; my strength, my fight...

I'm sorry my leaves fall frantically; in the search for wellness...

Leaving no apparent beauty; just diseased mass...

I am afraid that time is running out for my search...

Just little "signals" here and there...

   masses of magical elixirs...

Still the disease lies latent; the Greens ready to pounce their prey...

   spring-loaded...

The pain to my trunk; the damage still unknown...

I just want my life back my; beautiful wind...

I want to dance with you as you exhale...

I want to laugh with you...

Mmmm, love on you...

I know my leaves have fallen...

but; my beautiful wind...

Do I not have anymore; beauty that you can see?

In the times I have been steadfast waiting for a pocket of you to breeze by...

In my love and admiration...

That its unwavering and I stay grounded of it?

My essence is still here oozing out the cracks in my body...

Sometimes it takes looking up close and personal; to see the beauty bubbling...

   strength building...

It takes leaning on me to feel me; to get to know me...

How I am every time we are together...

That I am quiet, loving, strong, and can "dance" with you, even during sickness...

Seasons come and go...

I have understood and waited; through sickness and fighting this alone...

Is there not strength and beauty in this...

Even the strongest tree my great wind; will fall...

especially in the midst of constant turbulence...

She is salvageable; during a terrible season...

With a little touch and watering; the voice I imagine all plants crave...

She just needs to get away from it all...

To not be a diseased tree in a lone meadow...

And to fly away with you; light, free, healed.

Sometimes, I feel like diving head first into the "green waters"; let the angry waves pull me down…

The sea sickness sometimes too much to bear; so much so, I myself am green as they…

The angry waves from the depth of the green sea pull me to and fro; tug of war…

I wish to let go; so, I can live.

Communion

This is my body; not as it was before…

Yet I am still woman; and need you upon me…

Trace me with your fingers slowly; cleanse me…

These are my lips; Let me drink of your wine…

Feed me your body; so that I might be whole again.

The constant carousel; no ringed prize…

Viewed as crazy, lazy; no one knows…

My courage for fighting; goes unnoticed…

Sometimes, I can feel "The Greens" crawling through me…

Alive; yet I am six feet under…

Breathless; suffocating…

Energetic heart; yet exhaustion…

When will it stop, this hell that I am in; if ever?

After Thoughts from OZ

The subconscious mind is a very powerful thing. Numerous studies have been performed and theories proven on the subliminal effects of different music and the effects it has on the body. Earlier I am sure you noticed my reference to the music from Ghetto Boys. I am going to tell you something right now…that was some of the worst "herxing" I had gone through. Very close to the ABX.

I am sure you are wondering what in the world, made me try this. One day, after cussing and swearing at "my Lyme" as if it were an entity in front of me; i just had a light bulb thought…and ya' all will probably think I am crazy. LOL. There is scientific proof of this however.

I was feeling pretty, okay; that day I tried this. I thought it'd be funny to listen to that song from "Office Space" …and just like fuck you Lyme. LOL. Just listen. There was a study out of Japan and a book written about the study of water and our bodies and what just our thoughts do to water. Our bodies are about 60% water. So, if any negative thought etc. music can affect it. So, I tried it. What have I got to lose? Eh?

It might not totally be out of the realm of possibility, that we could purify our blood though killing them with songs about Back up in yo' ass with the resurrection...until we have no "herxing" after listening to it then turn it around and Mozart it. Just saying…and…

I was feeling good until that song. LOL! I felt like I was "herxing". Not only was I "herxing" but it was like "herxing" on crack! I listened to it a lot. Our bodies are very powerful. Wouldn't that be a kick in the fucking crotch, if it was killing off some of the bacteria. This "herxing" lasted about a week. It was pretty, severe.

Wouldn't that be a kick in the crotch? (Fuck yes I love that phrase! Thank you, Jennifer Anniston,!) If we could break this bacteria; down by listening to certain music making them weak so we could then kill the bacteria totally with our meds etc. If our bodies are 60% water that is a leg up. Means more control. We are the shareholders.

If we made 60% of our bodies a toxic pool for them to swim in, perhaps they'll die? The fucks, and our plasma...is 92% water. 55% of our blood volume...again more stock.

Dare to consider anything for your health. Just because one thing works for one person might not work for you. Don't get discouraged though just keep trying. You will find something. I know you will.

Other Things to Help You Through:

Don't give up everything pleasurable. Have the Danish, bread, wine, beer in moderation. It's a shit ass disease…and a luck of the draw anyway with Lyme. One day it will bother you next it won't. So, you might as well see…and feel semi-normal for a day. Do something that makes you feel sexy. Sexy is good helps us feel invincible.

Whether it's a sexy lipstick, panties, pedicures or dirty magazines. Just do it and; find someone to fight for and keep them as your focus point while you birth your health.

The thing I wish I would have done but didn't know about was have a natural health regimen ready for after the ABX. Taking things to calm and relax the body during this process. Take the anti-biotics for a longer period than three weeks which docs don't want to do then immediately as you go off start a hefty naturopath approach according to what you feel your body can handle.

Drink energized water. Pick some quartz crystal or other stones you feel your body needs. It completely changes the molecular structure of the water.

Take care of your soul. Baby it, and treat it as a treasure.

After what we have all gone through, I think we all need to petition that all MDs and FNP must take a specialty class related to Lyme, for a bill to be passed that insurance companies must pay for treatment and testing no matter how many, or how expensive, as well as regulations placed on LLMDs and the amount they can charge for their service. Also, regulations in place that any regular MD who denies someone help for the reason of Lyme is at risk for paying a fine as well as coming before the medical board. I was denied by so many; because and to their own statement: "I just don't know enough about it." Really? You are a doctor. It is your responsibility as a physician so stay up on this stuff. Period. I was denied by at least twenty LLMDs because I couldn't pay their fee. Many others, were denied help with insurance and forced to charge and spend their life savings just to get better. This is just wrong! We should also stand together as a community and appeal to our government wherever you live to start a separate funding; set up by our government specifically to help and treat Lyme.

I know some of you who have Lyme just want to roll over and die. DON'T Give up! There is help out there and lots of different things you can do to heal yourself.

Try to tickle your funny bone and have a laugh occasionally. Laughter is great medicine. Thank you, Impractical Jokers.

Do I do all these all the time NO! LOL. I forget and I am flawed like many of you. I do; however, try. When I do; do them…it helps and remember, those who can't do…teach!

I hope, that my book has educated you, made you laugh, and that it will continue to be an instrument for your healing. I realize for some I am that; "no thank you Maam". Others will be saying, "Oh yes give me some more Maam."

To all these variables of people I say I love you.

Thank you for being a most awesome part of my design...

And it begins....

Peace out, my lovelies.

In Love,

Nicolenya Caltman

References

The links provided were my favorite places to go, personally. Occasionally Facebook, but not a lot of support there to be honest because everyone is in their own misery with Lyme. There are a few people on there who are great and whose friendship I cherish. The one thing Facebook was good for was the articles people would post. So, just watch as they roll in. I wasn't really interested in all the Lyme sites that had news. I had Lyme, and that was news enough for me. I just wanted a cure, and to be surrounded by people who understood my fight. There weren't books I read because I had a very hard time reading as my brain was going. Most the books I looked at were dry. I would have loved an in your face book about it. This is why I wrote this.

I will say, it was very hard when sick; to search here and there and everywhere on the net for magical concoctions to work. There also wasn't just a one stop shop place. There will be soon.

For now, you can go to http://lymelyfe.pollywogbooks.com/ to watch for updates about the launch. Those of you wishing to contribute to the community email me as well as those suffering and needing support at: lymelyfe@pollywogbooks.com.

Links

https://www.lymedisease.org/lyme-basics/lyme-disease/about-lyme/

https://canlyme.com/living-with-lyme/

http://www.tiredoflyme.com/forum.html

https://www.youtube.com/results?search_query=neurological+lyme+disease

https://lymediseaseuk.com/

https://draxe.com/stevia-kills-lyme-disease/ Dr. Axe is a great reference! Has lots on Lyme.

http://lymecommunity.com/forums/ubbthreads.php/ubb/cfrm

https://www.lymeneteurope.org/forum/

https://thetickslayer.com/forum/

https://www.iherb.com/

https://www.swansonvitamins.com/

https://www.vitacost.com/

Ebay

Amazon

https://www.puritan.com/

http://www.naturalhealthlabs.com/deer-antler-spray

https://www.near-death.com/reincarnation/experiences/mellen-thomas-benedict.html

Above all my darlings; LOVE YOURSELVES…and know I LOVE YOU TOO!

FIN…and to be continued…